TREATMENT OF COMMON DISEASES WITH QI GONG THERAPY

Chief Editor
Li Xiang Ming,Yan Shan
Translator
Yu Min, Lu Xiao Zhen
Wang Fang, Lin Huan Ying

Academy Press [Xue Yuan]

First Edition 1997
ISBN 7 – 5077 – 0111 – 5/R·22

TREATMENT OF COMMON DISEASES WITH QI GONG THERAPY

Chief Editor: Li Xiang Ming, Yan Shan
Translator: Yu Min, Lu Xiao Zhen
Wang Fang, Lin Huan Ying

Published by
Academy Press [Xue Yuan]
11 Wanshoulu XiJie, Beijing 100036, China
Distributed by
China International Book Trading Corporation
35 Chegongzhuang Xilu, Beijing 100044, China
P.O. Box 399, Beijing, China

Printed in the People's Republic of China

FOREWORD

This book was written and edited, at the request of vast numbers of Qigong enthusiasts, by the famous Qigong master Li Xiangming while he was writing the book Genuine Qigong — the Three Treasures Supreme Harmony Qigong.

Li Xiangming, is the creator of Three Treasures Supreme Harmony Qigong, who has been practing Qigong for 30 years. As a doctor of Longevitiology, he was invited to participate in a large scale international seminar on medicine in Japan, where he delivered a speech on medical Qigong, which had attracted great deal of attention and appreciation from the participants who came from various parts of the world. In 1988 he was made an honorary member of the Association of International Natural Medicine. On 22, February 1990, a special program "Li Xiangming and Qigong" was broadcast on The China Central TV Station in its Program of "International Exchange".

The objective of this book is to enable Qigong

beginners as well as those who have a weak constitution or are in poor health to conduct some simple, practical and effective Qigong exercises, so as to have their illnesses relieved and to keep fit.

The Qigong therapy for common diseases provides Qigong amateurs with the methods for health and longevity. In the book, the basic principle of Qigong, including the requirements for Qigong practice, is introduced first. Then some common methods for keeping fit and for self-regulation, which are easy to learn and have been practiced by many Qigong amateurs, are provided. In order to facilitate the readers who want to relieve their disorders with the help of this book, some acupuncture points concerned with common diseases which are involved in Qigong practice and should be known are supplied in the latter part of the book. Qigong serves as a basis for elimination of disease. Conversely, good health promotes better Qigong practice.

May the book be of much help to our readers and Qigong amateurs!

editor

Acknowledgement

We gratefully acknowledge the contribution made by Mrs. Connie Beasley, an American medical specialist, to the correction of some parts of the English translation in the book.

CONTENTS

CHAPTER 1

CHAPTER 2

CHAPTER 1

I. Basic Principles of Qigong Practice

There are diverse schools and numerous Patterns of Qigong, which share some common points and similarities in regard to the basic principles.

In Qigong practice, no matter what mode is employed, lying, sitting, or standing, dynamic or static, it is required that the body postures assumed should be correct and comfortable throughout the entire practice. If the practitioner fails to adhere to correct body postures, the effect of Qigong exercise will not be obtained.

In conducting Qigong, the Qi and mind are interconnected, inter-dependent and inter-promoted. Qi is the essential substance of vital activity of the human body. It is also the basis for physiological functions of the viscera, meridians, organs and tissues. Therefore the major objective of Qigong practice lies in the training of Qi, during which, Qi inside the body is aroused to accumulate and guided to circulate along the meridians and collaterals. In the process of training Qi, the practioner should regulate his/her mind so as to make the body relaxed and to be in a natural state, the requirment of which is helpful in regulating Qi and blood and smoothing their circulation in the meridians and collaterals. In the practice, the interrelationship of mind and Qi, as well as the association of activity and tranquility are applied.

In Qigong circles, there are two opinions on mind exertion during Qigong practice. One opinion holds that the mind should be disregarded in the practice, which means that during the practice there is an absence of any thought in the mind of the practitioner, who should just be tranquil and relaxed. On the other hand, another opinion, believes in and stresses that the role of mind exertion is important in the practice. We think both opinions to certain extent are reasonable. Thus, they should be combined in Qigong practice.

As far as the Three Treasures Supreme Harmony Qigong is concerned, we advocate that in Qigong practice, the practitioner should not undergo strong mental exertion. For instance, in the practice, the practioner's mental attention on Dantian (Elixir Field) should not be intense. Once the Dantian region becomes warm and the intestines are peristaltic, let the Dantian region be free from attention and maintain it as it is.

In conducting Qigong practice, it is not appropriate to pursue high efficacy of Qigong after merely a short period of practice, such as forcing Qi to go through the "pass" i.e. "the small heavenly circuit" or "the large heavenly circuit", or opening the "heaven eye". If the practitioner is impetuous in Qigong practice, he/she may have an oppressed or suffocated feeling with dizziness, headache, palpitations, etc.. Therefore, the Supreme Harmony Qigong does not require strong mental exertion during the practice. The efficacy of Qigong will increase gradually as practice proceeds.

In Qigong practice, relaxation, tranqulization and being natural are of great significance. "Relaxation" means the whole body should be relaxed; "tranquilization" means keeping a peaceful mind; and "being natural" refers to the body postures and breathing being in a natural state, as well as keeping the mind free from forced exertion.

When the human body is in a relaxed state, the

consumption of oxygen decreases, the metabolic rate is reduced, much energy is stored, and there is good coordination between the sympathetic and parasympathetic nervous systems. These effects will further facilitate the regulation of Qi and blood, dredge the meridians and collaterals, and benefit the rectification and renovation of the organism so that health is promoted. In the practice, relaxation plays an important role in relieving the practitioner's mental stress, the limbs' and body's tension as well as obtaining the therapeutic effects of Qigong practice.

Thanquility of mind refers to a peaceful mental state, in which, there is not any stray thought in the mind disturbing the practitioner. The cerebral cortical function of tissues and organs of the whole body will thus be improved. Tranquility of the mind is, therefore very beneficial to the health, both physically and mentally.

Being natural includes natural body postures, natural and pleasant mental state and natural respiration. If the principle of being natural is observed in the practice, gradually there come the soreness, numbness, distension and warm sensations, which are known as "obtaining Qi". In addition, a creeping sensation, which may occur during Qigong practice suggests Qi circulating in the body, the phenomenon of which is also known as "Qi travelling". In fact, these sensations are not forced to appear by the practioner's subjective mental exertion, but present spontaneously as the practice proceeds.

Concerning the selection of a specific mode of Qigong practice, it is suggested that the practioner take his/her age, constitution and pathological condition into account so as to determine a proper mode of Qigong practice for him/herself. In the book some choices are offered to our practitioners in the chapter "Health Preservation Methods".

Undoubtedly, as there are great varieties of disease, one kind of Qigong is not suitable for all patients.

Ⅱ. Common Health Preserving Methods

Three common, practical, and simple modes of Qigong practice, namely, lying, sitting, and standing are offered here for beginners and weak persons or patients.

1. Lying

This method is applied in the evening or before sleep and is more suitable for weak persons, patients and old people. In the practice, the practitioner lies supinely with a thin pillow under the head, both arms lying at the sides of the body; the left palm of a male practitioner should face upward, the female's downward. The right palm of a male should lie against the bed; the female's should face upward (to take in the nature's Qi from heaven and earth). Meanwhile, the legs extend naturally with the feet shoulder-width apart, and the toes upward. The face and the five sense organs are relaxed, the mouth and the eyes shut naturally, and the practitioner is tranquil, free from stray thoughts. There should not be any one present near the practitioner, who should avoid being disturbed by a sudden sound.

2. Sitting

The practitioner sits either on a sofa, or a chair, or a bed with feet on the ground and shoulder-width apart, the knees flexed at a 90° angle, the thighs assuming a right angle with the trunk, the head and the neck; the hands are placed on the part of the thighs closer to the trunk, with palms facing upward. The thumbs and index fingers of each hand connect with each other. The shoulders are relaxed and elbows dropped; the chin is withdrawn slightly; the face of the practitioner is relaxed; the mouth and eyes are closed gently.

3. Standing

The practitioner stands with the feet shoulder-width apart, the toes forward. The knees are relaxed and slightly bent. The upper limbs hang at the sides of the body with hands relaxed and palms facing the legs; the chin is withdrawn a little; the mouth and eyes are closed naturally.

In conducting Qigong practice, the practitioner, depending on his/her physical condition, assumes one of the above three postures, then breathes in and out deeply once. Afterwards, a relaxed sensation of the body, including the internal organs is felt, the sensation of which has been mentioned before, and should be maintained throughout the entire exercise. Nevertheless, it is difficult for beginners to maintain the relaxed state for a long period of time. Usually, sometime later, tenseness of the body and an upward pulling sensation of the internal organs reappear. This phenomenon is considered to be normal in the initial practice, if relaxation of the body lasts merely a few minutes, take a few more deep breaths during the practice. Proceeding with the practice, the state of the practitioner will be transformed from the awkward to the normal. During the practice, while the body is relaxed, the practitioner should try as much as possible to get rid of stray thoughts from the mind, such as thinking about unaccomplished work, household affairs, or illness of the body, and enter into a tranquil state, ignoring self-existence. Failure to reach this state results in little effect from Qigong practice. It is recommended that Qigong exercise be conducted twice or three times daily, each time over twenty minutes. In the initial practice, however, it is better to do the exercise for a short period of time, then extend the time of training gradually as the health of the practitioner permits.

Haste should be avoided. In finishing the practice, remain in the same posture as assumed in the training. Open the eyes and rub the hands until the palms feel warm, the middle fingers rub respectively along the sides of nose from the ala nasi to the centre of the forehead, from where each middle finger travels laterally to the respective temple regions and goes downward along the cheeks. The massage is repeated 18 times; then, the practitioner slowly walks for a few minutes to complete the exercise. When the Qigong exercise is over, the practitioner feels pleasant and is entirely free from worry.

After one week or longer of exercise, the practitioner's palms will feel warm and distended during the practice. In addition, a numbness, tingling like mild electric current going through the fingers is experienced. The acupoint Yongquan (KI 1) located on the soles also feels warm, the toes distended and numb. This sensation is transmitted from the feet to the shanks, known as Qi sensation, which implies that the practitioner has "Qi".

Once there is Qi sensation, let the Qi flow inside the body. Meanwhile, gather the essential qi from nature, and dispel the pathogenic Qi from the body so as to achieve a curative effect.

Qi, which should not, however, be forced to move by mental exertion during Qigong exercise, flows in the body step by step, proceeding naturally; during practice, the flow of qi in various parts of the body is felt gradually and followed but not guided by the mind. One should not lead the Qi flow to any site of the body. On the contrary, the mind always goes behind the Qi flow. This is the key point of the Three Treasures Supreme Harmony Qigong training, which is derived from many years of experiences of Qigong Master Li Xiangming, Whose success in Qigong is dependent on it. Success for the practitioner of Qigong also results from it. If the pratitioner perseveres, Qigong deviation will be avoided.

It is proposed by someone that having reached a certain level of Qigong, efficacy will be realized, and the practitioner will be able to conduct Qigong so as to have Qi pass through the large and small heavenly circuits.

Health Preserving Qigong, however, stresses that the progress of Qigong practice from the simple to the difficult, such as conducting the Large Heavenly Circuit and the Small Heavenly Circuit Qigong, should proceed naturally, when Qi is trained to travel naturally in the whole body, the Qigong practice of allowing Qi to pass through the large and small heavenly circuits can be conducted so as to increase the efficacy of Qigong. The mind should not, however, be strongly focused on Qi circulation.

The term "heavenly circuit" used by ancient Qigong masters, refers to the passage of Zhenqi(Genuine qi) circulation, which is understood and explained differently by different schools of Qiong. Here, the term will not be explained as it is not much concerned with the Common Health Preserving Qigong. The following paragraphs will introduce Qigong of Clear Qi Inhalation (the essential Qi of heaven and earth), and dispelling Turbid Qi (the pathogenic Qi in the body).

Throughout the above mentioned practice, when the genuine Qi is obtained and circulates naturally in the body, the following methods of practice are conducted to get rid of the pathogenic Qi (turbid Qi) from the body for various disorders, so that the objective of healing and strengthening the body is achieved.

1. Taking in the Clear Qi and dispelling the turbid Qi

Guiding the clear Qi, (thinking the essential Qi coming from the heaven and the earth) to enter

Baihui(GV 20), from where it flows along the route of Jianjing (GB 21) — Danzhong (CV 17) — Zhongdantian (mid Elixir Field) — Huiyin (CV 1) — Yinlingquan (SP 9) — Sanyinjiao (SP 6) — Yongquan (KI 1) — the big toe — the second toe — the third toe — the fourth toe — the small toe then turning around the bottom of foot, back to Yongquan (KI 1), ascending from the lateral side of the foot — Yanglingquan (GB 34) — Huantiao (GB 30) — Changqiang (GV 1) — Mingmen (GV 4) — Zhongdantian (mid-Elixir Field) from where the Qi circulating downward and repeating the above mentioned circle.

2. Blood pressure reducing for hypertension

Assume either the lying or sitting posture in a relaxed state, concentrate the mind at Yongquan (KI 1). In the practice, the practitioner must be relaxed and concentrate on Dantian (Elixir Field) while breathing in, concentrate on Yongquan (KI 1) while breathing out. In this way Qi and blood descend, causing blood pressure to be reduced.

3. Rehibilitation for patients of cerebral vascular accidents with sequellae of limbs dysfunction.

Adopt the lying or sitting posture of Qigong exercise. After relaxing the body, concentrate the mind at Laogong (P 8) of the immobile hand and

Yongquan (KI 1) of the immobile leg, causing Qi to remove the obstruction in the meridians and collaterals on its way to circulating through these points to restore the normal functions of the extremities. Massage is also recommended to be applied frequently on the affected limbs.

III. Therapy of Qi Gathering and Emitting

Retarded flow of Qi or obstruction of Qi and blood circulation in the meridians and collaterals is the cause of a great variety of diseases. Qigong therapy enables the removal of Qi and blood obstruction from meridians and collaterals, thus, diseases are relieved.

The therapy of Qi Gathering and Emitting provides a way for the practitioner, who assists patients in the removal of Qi and blood obstruction from meridians and collaterals through emitting his/her Qi to the patients so that the purpose of rehibilitation will be achieved.

Methods:

1. The practitioner gathers his/her internal Qi to his/her Laogong (P 8) (located in the centre of the palm pointed by and between the tips of the middle and ring fingers when they are fully flexed). When the practitioner breathes out, his/her palms emit Zhen Qi (antipathogenic Qi) to the affeted site

or a relevant point of the patient, and the palms move 15-20cm away from the affected site or the point of the patient when the practitioner breathes in, in this way, the pathogenic Qi of the patient is obsorbed out of the body. The process is repeated 36 times.

2. A pain occuring in a certain site on a patient can result from obstruction of Qi and blood circulation in the meridians and collaterals. The practitioner emits Qi for a few minutes through his/her Laogong (P 8) point, which is kept 5 cm away to the affected site or a relevant point on the patient who concentrates his/her mind at Yong-quan (KI 1) to make the pathogenic Qi descend along the course of the meridian and flow out of Yongquan(KI 1).

3. The practitioner closes his/her thumb, fore-finger and the middle finger, at the tips of which internal Qi of the practitioner is transferred and emitted to the affected site or a relevant point on the patient. As the Qigong efficacy level of practitioners varies, acupoint pressing or massage can be supplemented.

4. The practitioner gathers his/her genuine Qi at Laogong (P 8), and his/her palms, which are then put on the pain site or a relevant point of the

patient. Press and turn in the direction from the medial to the lateral with moderate force 36 times. In this way the genuine Qi of the practitioner is transmitted to the patient, resulting in dispersing of Qi and blood stagnation at the affected site, and the pathogenic Qi is discharged out of the body through the course of meridians and collaterals.

The above explanations provide the practitioner with methods of emitting his/her genuine Qi to the patient, through which the pathogenic Qi of the patient is discharged out of the body. Nevertheless, if patients conduct Qigong exercise themselves and cooperate with the practitioner, the effect will be better, because patients change their positions in the treatment from the passive into the active which is an aim of the introduction of Qigong therapy.

If patients have knowledge of the relevant points used for the treatment of their disorders, they can apply massage on these points themselves or be massaged by family members, or treated with a magnetic device for self-preservation of health. In the later part of the book Qigong exercises for common diseases are introduced in detail.

IV. Methods for Self Regulation

In passing on Qigong skills, Master Li Xiangming often teaches people some practical Qigong
exercises which have been collected and sorted out
by him for years. Many Qigong amateurs and
patients have benefited from these Qigong exercises. Therefore, these exercises are offered in the
following paragraphs for those people who are
busily engaged in their work, do not have specific
time for exercise, are often troubled by some
malaise and eager to learn Qigong. They are
advised to select a suitable method of exercise from
the following based on their respective physical
conditions. It is hoped that they will profit from
the methods introduced herein.

1. On your way to work or home after work, or
when you go for a walk, concentrate the mind on
Baihui (GV 20) located on the vertex, Yongquan
(KI 1) in the soles and Laogong (P 8) in the palms,
relax the whole body as much as you can. This
makes your body communicate with the Qi of

nature and absorb the essential Qi from the heaven and the earth. Doing this you will feel your energy is increased while working, and your fatigue caused by your work is relieved. This method has the effect of strengthening the body and increasing work efficiency.

2. Assume the standing or sitting posture 10 to 15 minutes before working or studying, concentrate the mind on Baihui (GV 20) and Yongquan (KI 1) so as to take in the essential Qi from the heaven and the earth. The essential Qi which is taken in mixes with Qi in Shenque (CV 8) located in the navel and ascends to Laogong (P 8) located in the palms. This method makes you feel more energetic at the commencement of your work or study, and you will work more efficiently.

3. After getting up in the morning, comb your hair with your fingers from the anterior to the posterior of the head, then rub the hands till they become warm; afterwards, let the hands rub the face down 18 – 36 times. This method serves to prevent hair from early greying, reduce facial wrinkles and maintain youth.

4. Prior to sleep in the eveninng, lie on the bed, concentrate the mind on the same points mentioned in the second method so as to open the

points to take in the essential Qi from the nature; relax the whole body in order to get rid of the fatigue, and be tranquil. This method will result in a sound sleep.

The third method mentioned above which is quite beneficial for insomnia and neurasthenia patients can also be applied in the evening.

5. Think of the moon light or the clear light of the stars that enters Baihui (GV 20) located at the vertex where the clear light of the moon or stars turns into a line traveling to Yintang (EX – HN3) on glabella. At Yintang, the light divides into 2 branches going into Zanzhu (BL 2), the clear light then circulates around the orbit. This method can be adopted for eye disorders, such as styes, cataracts, conjunctivitis, near-sightedness, far-sightedness, weak sight in children, etc.

6. Before work or study, sit up straight with palms facing each other. Push the palms toward each other and pull them back to their respective sides to draw Qi. When sensation of Qi is felt between the hands, join the hands together and put them on Dantian (Elixir Field) located in the lower abdomen below the navel. Close the eyes to calm down the mind with the attention focused on Dantian and the spirit on Zuqiao (3 cun deep inside

Yintang, the glabella). Enter the Qigong state and maintain it for some 10 minutes. Afterwards, start work or study. The practitioner will be full of vigor and have a clear mind, sharp thinking and improved memory. This exercise can be conducted before sleep in the evening for neurasthenia, insomnia, etc.

7. Stand naturally with the body in a fully relaxed state, put the thumbs, fore-fingers, and middle fingers of both hands, which connect with each other, on the navel, cover the bilateral Tianshu (ST 25) located laterally to the navel by Laogong (P 8) located in the palms. In this way the lower abdomen feels warm with the sensation of Qi flowing in the abdomen. Twenty minutes later, the medial side of both elbows firmly touch the ribs, then the middle finger, whose tips possess the point Zhongchong (H 1) press the bilateral Qichong (ST 30) located at the upper end of thighs. Moreover, the palms, which are firmly against the upper end of the thighs, conduct massage in a backward direction. This method is applied for Yang deficiency with aversion to cold and irregular menses.

8. Assume the standing posture as required in Qigong exercise with palms upward and middle finger tips connecting with each other; separate

the other fingers naturally, relax the shoulders and elbows; keep both hands at the level of the navel; close the eyes, think about the state of being in the shower with fine streams of water flowing from the head down to the shoulders, the body, and the feet, and then entering the ground. The water in the palms goes down through the fingers to the ground. This method has the effect of reducing blood pressure.

9. Assume the standing posture. The body is relaxed with arms hanging naturally at the sides. Concentrate the mind on bilateral Hegu (LI 4) located on the hands; rotate the hands lightly backward. This practice causes peristalsis of the intestines and the desire to empty the bowels. This method is beneficial for old people with a constipation problem.

10. Adopt the standing posture; relax the whole body. Let the tongue lap against the outside of the front teeth; stretch the neck to relax the nape. This method reduces the malaise of cervical spondylopathy.

11. Assume the standing posture; relax the whole body; roll up the tongue. This method prevents and heals urticaria.

12. Assume the standing or sitting posture.

Slightly close the eyes; relax the body naturally; rub hands to make them warm; separate the fingers and comb the hair 36 times. Afterwards, both hands press the scalp, kneading and rubbing the scalp towards the vertex 36 times, then knead and rub from the sides to the back 36 times. Finally, tap the scalp gently with finger tips 18 times.

This method prevents hair falling and early greying.

13. Assume the sitting posture as required in Qigong exercise. Massage the ears and the mastoid regions with fingers of both hands 24-36 times. Pinch and pull the auricle 24-36 times; press with the finger Yifeng (TE 17). Tinggong (SI 19), Wangu (GB 12) for 1 minute respectively. This method is applied twice daily in the morning and in the evening. It is helpful for improving hearing and nerve deafness.

14. Adopt the sitting posture, close the eyes and hold the breath. Cover your ears with your hands, with the fingers knocking the occiput (beating the heavenly drum) 36 times. This method is applied for dizziness and headache.

15. Assume the standing posture; hold the head with both hands; move the body forward, back-ward, left and right 30 times. It is good to induce

sweating through the exercise. This method is applied twice daily for blurred vision, deafness, and headache.

16. Adopt either the standing or sitting posture; hold the mandibles up by both hands; hold the breath till the mouth feels numb. Afterwards, be relaxed and knock the teeth 36 times. This method is conducted 5 times daily for toothache.

17. Assume the standing or sitting posture, open the eyes wider; breath in 9 mouthful Qi continously; let the mind and Qi reach Dantian (Elixir Field).

This method is applied for bleeding nose.

18. Adopt the sitting posture, rub the palms till they become warm; massage the waist and the knees 36 times, the method of which is used for pain of the low back and legs. For severe cases, the massage is increased.

19. Assume the sitting posture with both hands lying gently on the Dantian (Elixir Field) located below the navel, this method which increases the warmth inside the abdomen is applied for the treatment of abdominal pain.

20. Stand as required in the Qigong exercise. Hold the breath and turn the body left and right, then change both hands into fists, one fist rises and

the other goes down. This movement is applied alternately and respectively 21 times. It is conducted for abdominal distention and dyspepsia.

V. Methods of Health Preservation and Longevity

Though there are various ways to preserve health and prolong life, the essential ways will not stray from the word "quiescence," "Huang Di Yin Fu Jing" (Huang Di's Classic of Yin Figures) says:" The law of nature is quiescence, which ensures the birth of all things in heaven and earth." Taoists often believe that "Quiescence is the gate of birth, while movement is the door of death," "Zhi Guan" (quiet watch) and "Chan Ding" (meditation) in Buddhism are the methods set up to practise and pursue quiescence. Maintenance of quiescence not only leads to fitness and disease resistance, but also prolongs life and promises longevity. Quiescence may bring about stability, which in turn gives birth to wisdom. Freguent practice of charitable and pious deeds may lead to a supreme state where the mind is purified, and the temperament cultivated, things follow their own courses, heaven and men are in harmony.

Ancient saints have left us a lot of instructions in relation to " Health Preservation". Those who paid attention to health preservation must have highly valued their lives; those who highly valued their lives must have underestimated material wealth. Never sacrifice one's body for desire, nor sacrifice one's conscience for fame, nor sacrifice one's life for profit. Keep the inside and outside apart, and keep the inside and outside quiet. Forget both the inside and outside so as to enter a state of being purified, empty, quiet and stable, which promises natural longevity and the progress of comprehension with wisdom. That is the law of nature.

Ⅰ. **Methods to train the mind**

1. Formula of the character "Forget":

To forget material wealth to cultivate the mind; to forget emotion to cultivate the temperament; to forget circumstances to replenish the mind; to forget sex to nourish the essence; to forget oneself to tonify the deficiency; to forget everything and then everything is strengthened.

2. Formula of the character "Light hearted":

It's better to care less fame, profit, desire, sex, and love, to be less angry, suspicious or competitive. If one is light-hearted, then there is always peace.

3. Formula of the character "Less":

Speak less to save qi; Watch less to promote hearing; Ask less to cultivate temperament; Think less to protect the heart; Gain less to preserve essence; Move less to replenish the mind; "Being (or achieving) less leads to clarity."

4. Formula of character "Quiescence":

The physigue should be still, the mind calm, and qi quiet. During Qigong practice, tranquility is required not only in the process of practising qigong, but also at ordinary times. Try to search for quiescence within both tranguility and noise. Quiescence promotes stability and stability gives birth to wisdom.

5. Formula of the character "Little":

Little essence should be discharged; little energy should be consumed; little qi should be lost; One should enjoy less happiness, seek less fame, accumulate less profit. Moreover, less worry promotes more spirit.

6. Formula of the character "Nothing", or "No":

Facing the view, but there is no view; Living in the world, but there is no world; Intending to think, but there is no thought; Concentrating the mind, but there is no mind. Nothing exists, no heaven, no earth, no people, not even oneself. The genius of Taoism is to train the mind to reveal the void, to train the void to reveal nothing. Buddhism requires unconciousness of the body's outward appearance, unconciousness of oneself, all living creatures and Buddhists; unawareness of the eye, ear, nose, tongue, body and mind, as well as unawareness of color, sound, smell, taste, feeling and ways. In a word, the greatest attainments of Buddhism and Taoism can be summarized by the character "Nothing".

7. Formula of the character "Good":

To cultivate good temperament, to be good-hearted, to practice good deeds, to treat others well, to persuade others to do good, to be good both inside and outside, to have both moral integrity and conduct. If everyone does good, evil will no longer exist, the country will be peaceful, and people safe.

8. Formula of the character "Heart":

All methods stem from the heart, all ways stem from the heart. The heart is man's authority, governor of essence, qi and mind. Essence manufacture, qi practice and mind training all depend on cultivation of the heart first. The heart includes both motion and quiescence. If the heart remains motionless, there will be emptiness and quiescence and a display of the original human nature. One may forget himself mentally and physically. There is no heart within his heart. Unawareness of the heart is the Tao. In order to check one's desire, the inducing factors should be removed. Nothing can enter from the outside, nothing can be produced inside.Close oneself to external contact (namely, color, sound, smell, taste, feeling and ways), and to the internal six roots (namely, eye, ear, nose, tongue, heart and mind). Then, facing up to the heart again, it is calm in the face of wealth, desire, life and death. Being calm is close to the Tao.

9. Formula of the character" Preserve":

Less speaking preserves internal qi, less sex preserves essence and qi, light taste preserves blood and qi; Swallowing of saliva preserves Zang qi, restraining anger preserves liver qi, control of diet preserves stomach qi; Even fetus breathing preserves lung qi, less thinking preserves heart qi, less leakage of essence preserves kidney qi, careful behavior preserves vital qi.

10. Formula of the character "Morality":

Lao Zi said:" Morality brings back the state of infancy." For prolonging life and returning to youth, one must never be away from morality. One should put other's interest ahead of his own; treat others kindly but himself simply; attribute a fault to himself, but success to others; Don't stubbornly persist in one's own opinions, nor be self-satisfied and deny others. Never play up one's own by playing down others, flaunt one's superiority to show off, bully others because of the strength of a powerful position, behave arrogantly, or utter slander about others. One should earn his own living, cultivate himself to redeem lost souls by making offerings and saying prayers. One should not rob nor cheat others out of their money, nor practise graft. If he can accept both the sweet and bitter, be kind-hearted and honest, cultivate himself all the time, hold his beliefs persistently, he may surely return to the state where the nature of everything is revealed.

II. Methods of health preservation:

1. Diet should be proper: Don't eat and drink too much at one meal, don't limit oneself to one variety of food, don't eat between meals, don't overeat. Eat less hot and spicy food, or meat and fish, but more vegetables and fruits.

2. Daily life should be regular: It is good to go to bed early and get up early, to work and rest

according to a schedule; Neither stay up late, nor sleep too much.

3. Physical exercises should be combined with proper rest:

One should do physical labour, but within the limitation of fatigue; select some favorable recreational activities, such as listening to traditional opera, light music, or growing flowers, etc. Don't spend too much time playing chess or cards because prolonged concentration on them takes up one's energy.

4. Movement should be integrated with quiescence:

Movement and quiescence are opposite in nature. But once they are integrated, they are on the one hand opposite and on the other hand unified. They supplement and complement each other. Body movement builds up health, while mind tranquility keeps sufficient qi.

5. Air should be fresh:

The breath of heaven and earth, mountain and water, flower and plants is closely linked and associated with human beings, which benefits people greatly (except a few trees and plants which are poisonous). So, people should often go out to take a walk or practise qi gong. The room should be well ventilated.

6. Reading and watching should be properly controlled:

Prolonged reading or watching consumes energy. Consumption of energy disperses qi. Dispersing of qi results in blood deficiency which leads to blurred vision and dizziness. So, reading and entertainment should be controlled and done in proper hours.

7. The state of mind should be cheerful:

One should have a light heart, be happy in a good mood. Being in a cheerful state of mind is the basis of practising Qigong and prolonging life. A Chinese saying says:"A good laugh makes you ten years younger." One should be broadminded, open and aboveboard, holding no extravagant hopes because contentment always brings happiness.

8. Anger should be cleared away:

Anger, loss of temper and being narrow-minded are in conflict with health preservation. Sun simiao said:"Frequent anger disturbs joints all over the body," Hui nanzi said," Anger injures yin." Qi is stirred when yin is injured, the mind is absent when the heart is disturbed, the body is invaded by pathogenic qi when the mind is absent. This gives rise to various diseases. Therefore, people should be calm and even tempered, deal with things peacefully, check anger to preserve yin for the growth of qi.

9. The desire of greed should be eliminated

If a person is greedy with the desire for fame, profit, power, joy, drinking and sex, he may try every means to reach his aims at the expense of others, taking graft, embezzling, or murdering. He cares nothing for discipline, laws, regulations, and traditional morality. Longing for desires consumes heart qi, consumption of heart qi leads to absent mind. "Tai Xi Jing" (Classic of Fetus Breathing) says:"There is birth when qi is infused into the body, and there is death when the mind goes away from the body". So, Buddhists put "Greediness" in the first place. The desire of greediness should be eliminated. The mind should be calm and peaceful. That is a rare treasure for health preservation.

10. For health preservation, people need to have a high aspiration:

The confucianists emphasize that to cherish a high aspiration. Zhang heng-qu said:"One should be determined to serve heaven, earth, and living creatures. Hui neng, the sixth founder of Buddhism said:"Living creatures are determined to redeem lost souls by making offerings and saying prayers to be free from endless affliction." Tian xuanzi, a Toaist said:"The way of self cultivation is boundless, heaven and earth are immeasurable, so, one must mend his ways.In practising Qigong, we also need to have a great aspiration:"to benefit people". With a great aspiration, a noble spirit is aroused naturally. One is able to face up to himself and communicate with heaven and earth." Truth is derived from the heart. Laws are generated from the heart." With such an aspiration and determination, one is able to share morality with heaven and earth, share brightness with the sun and moon. His aspiration and determination will be in harmony with the universe. He may enter a supreme state of unity between heaven and man, where nothing exists in the heart,and the heart remains pure, and the nature of everything is revealed. This state is not only limited to health preservation and longevity, it leads to a way for communication between heaven and man.

III. Methods of longevity

1. Static Qigong

Static Qigong includes precious methods of health preservation handed down from our ancestors. Yin Fu Jing (Classic of Yin Figures), says:"The law of nature is quiescence, which gives rise to the growth of everything. Lao Zi advocated, "To reach the extreme void and keep quiet." Yan Zi insisted on "Zuo Wang"(sitting forgetfully), buddhism holds"Zhi Guan"(watching quietly) and "Chan Ding"(Meditation), all of which demand "quiescence". Quiescence can bring about stability, and stability gives birth to wisdom. In a narrow sense, meridians and collaterals can be activated, genuine qi tonified, digestive organs strengthened, blood circulation promoted, kidney functions consolidated, nerve systems perfected, psychosomatic functions regulated, metabolism speeded up, immune functions improved, diseases removed naturally, and life prolonged. In a broad sense, qi is replenished, essence nourished, morality cultivated, mind calmed, wisdom accumulated. A supreme state of harmony between heaven and man, and the presence of original human nature is promised.

Method of sitting still to communicate with both the heaven and earth: knee—crossing posture (single, double or natural knee-crossing) Relax the whole body, close the eyes gentlly. The head faces to the front, the spinal column is kept straight. Get .rid of all disturbing thoughts, calm the heart and concentrate the mind. Formula: Accumulate yin essence, knock Di Hu (the door of earth), rise to the hall, and enter the room; collect the sun light, enter the middle jiao, associate water with fire. Keep a hand gesture (two plams facing up, with the left hand on the right hand, resting below the umbilicus). Connect two thumbs gentlly, close the eyes, watching and listenning to the interior reactions. Imagine oneself sitting on a lotus stand, surrounded by abundant clean water, with many spots of blue light knocking Di Hu (Hui Yin, CV1). Look at Di Hu interiorly. When Di Hu Starts to shake or turn, concentrate the mind on absorbing the blue light. infusing it into the body gently, ascending at the lower "Dantian" through the central vessel. Then, close Di Hu, imagine once more that there are lots of white light spots in the sky, pronounce "Weng" in silence, let the white light to descend at the lower "Dantian" through the central vessel from" Tian Men" (Xingmen). So, yin qi of the earth and yang qi of the heaven can meet kidney water and heart fire at the lower "Dantian". Ba Gua (The Eight Diagramme after birth) holds that the umbilicus is the certral Wu Ji Tu, "middle jiao".

Repeat the process 36 times and then stop, to concentrate on the lower "Dan-tian" and look at upper "Dantian" interiorly. when umbilicus wheel, chest wheel, head wheel all stop turning, the heart becomes void, abdomen full, concentration relaxed. There is no more desire, thoughts, worries and fear. Focusing on the center of "∴" arranged only by the left eye, the right eye or Tian Mu, and looking at the middle and lower "Dantian" interiorly, all the disturbing thoughts of the whole life stop. Continuous practice may lead to a state of "dead heart but living mind".

While sitting still, it is possible to have some scence in the front. Don't "receive" the good ones, nor "be afraid of" those fierce ones. If there is no scence being seen, do not seek to have it. If one can keep on practising, he can enter a joyful world where the original nature of things is revealed.

2. Dynamic Qigong

Get rid off all disturbing thoughts. Keep a standing posture with relaxation and tranquility; Be in a good mood with smile. Form a hand gesture (the thumb tip being against the palmar side of the root of the ring finger, the other four fingers covering the thumb to make a fist by flexion) and put the two fists on the hypochondrium, turn the body to the left, step forward to the left with the left foot, move the body weight to the right foot, smile with the face turning up to the left.

Concentrate the mind on breathing "inhale-inhale-exhale" rhythmatically, at the same time, knock the ground 3 times gently with the heel of the left foot, and tap Shen-shu (BL 23) 3 times with the dorsal side of the left fist, Tianshu (ST 25) 3 times with the plamar side of the right fist. Then, turn the body to the right, step forward to the right with the right foot, move the body weight to the left foot, smile with the face turning up to the right. Concentrate the mind on breathing" inhale-inhale-exhale", at the same time, knock the ground 3 times gently with the heel of the right foot, and tap Tian-shu (ST 25) 3 times with the palmar side of the left fist, and shen-shu (BL 23) 3 times with the dorsal side of the right fist. Such alternation is just like walking in a garden at ease and peacefully. A person is away from restrictions and worries.

This Qigong technique is simple but with a profound theoretical basis, and qicek efficacy. In the selection of points, Tianshu (ST 25) is an important point of the Stomach Meridian of Foot Yangming, as well as the Front-Mu point of the Large Intestine Meridian of Hand Yangming, "Gui Gu Zi" says:" Tianshu in the body is in close relations to the germination, growth, transformation and storage. " Tianshu in the sky is the big Dipper, it is the center for the movement of other stars. In the human body, it is the center for transportation of the Umbilicus Diagramme; where qi ascends and descends, water and food are transported and transformed, it is a key point for the physiological functions of the whole digestive systems. Though Shenshu (BL 23) is a point of the Urinary Bladder Meridian of Foot Taiyang, it connects with the kidney interiorly. So it is the place where the essential qi of the kidney is infused. "Zhen Jiu Da Cheng" (Great Compendium of Acupuncture and Moxibustion) written by Yang Jizhou in the Ming Dynasty, points out:"Shenshu (BL 23) is indicated for emaciation of a consumptive syndrome, deafness and tinnitis due to kidney deficiency ⋯ low back pain, XiaoKe syndrome (diabetis), and five strains and seven impairments, and edema. In this Qigong, gentle and regular tapping on Tianshu (ST 25) and Shenshu (BL 23) can not only invigorate the qi and blood circulation in the meridians and collaterals, but also tonify the kidney and build up the spleen. The kidney which dominates essence, is the congenital foundation, while the spleen which dominates transformation of food is the aquired fundation. The regulation on both the congenital and aquired strengthens the Zang Fu organs and replenishes qi and essence. In addition, knocking the ground with heels promotes the communication of the three yang meridians of foot with three yin meridians of foot, and the smooth flow of qi and blood. Breath concentration increases the vital capacity, speeds up exhaling the old and inhaling the new and gas exchange, and strengthens the immunological functions of the respiratory system. The rhythmic turning of the head, neck, low back and knees to both the left and right side has a good therapeutic effect on relieving scapulohumeral periarthritis, rheumatic and rheumatoid arthritis, vertebral hyperplasia and retrogressive disorders, pain and motor impairment due to trauma and injury.

In a word, this Qigong practice requires a happy mood, and regulates the body functions both mentally and physically. Through tonifying the spleen and kidney, the functions of the five zang and six fu organs are strengthened and functional activities promoted. Breath concentration can activate the qi activites of ascending, descending, emerging and entering the body to improve the normal process of matabolism, thus, ensuring harmony among heaven, earth and man, simutaneous activities of mind, qi and body, balance of yin and yang, and free flow of qi and blood. Therefore, there remains no space for the invasion of pathogenic qi, no source for occurrence of diseases. How couldn't one have a long life?

Key points to practise this Qigong are as follows:

1)Be in a good and joyful mood. Imagine that you are having a walk among flowers and trees, or on a boulevard, with a feeling that the world is so beautiful and life is so happy. Never be jealous of others, nor expect what you can not get, if you practise Qigong, you can really understand the meaning of the Saying:"Buddhist patriarch never has worries in mind; and celestial being never has diseases in body."

2)Keep a hand gesture (Jin Gang Ying) all the time. "Jin Gang Ying" is termed by Buddhism, the Confucianism and Taoism call it "Wo Gu" (clench fist). The fetus in his mother's abdomen is clenching his fist like this till his birth. A chapter about health preservation, physical and breathing exercises in "Zhu Bing Yuan Hou Lun" (General Treatise on the Causes and Symptoms of Diseases) written by Chao Yuanfang in the Shui Dynasty says:" Qi will not leak, if one clenches his fist in the way a baby does." "Yang Xing Yan Ming Lu" (Records on Cultivation and Longevity) Wirtten by Tao Hongjing in the Southern Dynasties points out," If one can keep on clenching his fist, pathogenic qi and all toxic factors have no way to enter the body, essence will be strengthened, and eyes brightened, long life promised. " So, to make a hand gesture (Jin Gang Ying) can not only prevent essential qi in the body from being dispersed, but also avoid the disturbance to the mind by bad information from the external world. It can calm the mind, tranquilize thinking and lead to a state of Qigong naturally.

3)Being far sighted, one should turn his body freely, naturally and flexibly.

4)The breathing sound from the nose, "inhale-inhale-exhale" orders the palmar side of the fist to tap Tianshu (ST 25), dorsal side of the fist to tap Shenshu (BL 23) and heel to knock the ground respectively 3 times. They should be performed simutaneously with happiness, relaxation and the rhythm of a waltz.

5)Selection of points should be accurate. Tian shu (ST 25) is 2 cun lateral to the umbilicus, Shenshu (BL 23) is 1.5 cun lateral to Mingmen (GV 4). The two points are located in opposition. While tapping Tianshu (ST 25) in the front or Shenshu (BL 23) on the back, one should tap the point on the same side, never exceed the anterior or posterior midline.

3.Methods to communicate with heaven and tonify yang Qi:

Assume a standing posture with the feet shoulder-width apart. Stand in a relaxed and tranquilized state.

1) Collecting yang from the frontal side:

Lift the two arms from both sides gently, with palms facing up; Imagine that th plam is at the same level with the sky. Try to collect the white light from the sky into Laogong (PC 8) and Shixuan (tips of the ten fingers) as much as possible. Raise the palms gradually. when the palms are full of qi, raise them further above the vertex, infuse the white light to Tian Men (Life Pass) Then, put the palms together, moving downward along the anterior midline. While pronouncing" Weng", concentrate the mind on conducting the white light to the lower Dantian along the central vessel, and squat down. Along with the movement of collecting the white light again with the plams, the body ascends gradually. Repeat the whole process 9 times.

2) Turning the body to the left and collecting yang:

Turn the body halfway forward to the left. Lift the two palms from both sides, collect the white light, and move the body weight to the front. Lift the right heel from the ground slowly; When the palms reach the superior aspect of the vertex, infuse the white light to Tian Men (Life Pass). Put the palms together, and concentrate the mind on conducting the white light to the lower Dantian along the central vessel while pronouncing "Weng". At the same time, sit back, and lift the tip of the left foot from the ground slowly. Repeat the process 9 times.

3) Turning the body to the right and collecting yang:

Turn the body forward to the right. Lift the two palms from both sides, collect the white light, move the body weight to the front, lift the left heel from the ground slowly. When the palms reach the superior aspect of the vertex, infuse the white light to Tian Men (Life Pass). Put the palms together, concentrate the mind on conducting the white light to the lower Dantian along the central vessel while pronouncing "Weng". At the same time, sit back, and lift the tip of the right foot from the ground slowly. Repeat the process 9 times.

4) Collecting yang to infuse the brain:

Return to the standing posture again. Collect the white light from two sides with the hands. Infuse it into Tian Men, pronounce "Weng" once more, turn the palms, running down along the central vessel. Concentrate the mind on conducting the white light down to the lower Dantian. Then, lift the right plam (facing up) to collect white light. While pronouncing "Weng", infuse the white light into the head along Tian Men. Meanwhile, sway the head, waist and hips to the right. Move the body weight to the right; Successively, lift the left palm to collect white light while pronouncing "weng". Infuse the white light into the head along Tian Men. Meanwhile, sway the head, waist and hips to the left. Move the body weight to the left. Repeat the process on the right and left 9 times. Then, put the palms together, moving down slowly along the Conception Vessel, conducting qi to the lower Dantian. Finally, the palms droop naturally on the lateral sides of the thighs.

The name of this qigong exercise is called "communicating with heaven and tonifying yang qi". In this Qigong practice, a person is able to communicate with heaven with the aid of pronouncing "weng", and to collect miraculous qi to tonify yang qi in the body. A chapter of Nan Jing (Classic on Medical Problems) points out:"Qi is the root of a man. If the root is dead, the stems and leaves will be withered." Qi pertains to yang, and is marked by movement. So. it is also called "Yang Qi". It is the essential substance and energy that maintains the life activities of the body. If yang qi is deficient, there will be such symptoms as shortness of breath, dislike of speaking, general lassitude, poor appetite, low spirit caused by weak motivation, or aversion to cold and cold limbs, clear urine and loose stools due to deficiency of heat energy, or frequent attacks of common cold, sweating after exertion due to weakness of defens-ive qi in the exterior, scanty urine, puffiness, impairment of qi circulation due to failure of qi activities, purpura, epistaxis, hematuria and bloody stools due to heat in blood. So, those who have the above mentioned qi deficiency syndromes, should practise Qigong more. Yang qi in the body can be promoted through communicating with heaven. Once yang qi is tonified, diseases can be cured naturally, people become stronger and are full of vigor.

key points to practise this Qigong:

1)Give full play to the functions of pronouncing "Weng". It can not only improve the efficacy of collecting yang, but also promote the communication of yang in the lower Dantian;

2)Move the body upward and downward naturally in harmony while collecting the white light. Move the body straight up and slowly. While conducting the white light to the lower Dantian, squat down slowly with ease;

3)Keep the spinal column straight all the time. When the body is turned to collect yang, move the body weight forward without bending the waist. When sitting back, never throw out the abdomen.

4.Methods to communicate with the earth and benefit yin:

1) Obtaining yin from the frontal side:

Follow the previous posture. Hold the ground with ten toes gently, move the two hands backward from the lateral sides of the body with the palms facing down, and push forward slowly. Concentrate the mind on absorbing the blue light at the deep root of the ground to Yongquan (KI 1), Laogong (PC 8) and Shixuan (Extra). Move the body upward slowly while pronouncing "Hong". Pull the palms backward slowly, concentrate the mind on conducting the blue light abtained from Yongquan (KI 1) along the medial sides of the thighs through Di Hu (Perinium) to the lower Dantian; conduct the blue light obtained from the palms to the lower Dantian along the medial sides of the arms through the central vessel. At the same time, squat down gradually. Repeat the process 7 times.

2) Turning the body to the left and obtaining yin:

Turn the body forward to the left. Push forward slowly with the palms to collect the blue light. Move the body weight forward. Lift the right heel from the ground slowly. While pronouncing " Hong", pull the palms backward slowly, concentrate the mind on conducting the blue light to the lower Dantian along the central vessel. At the same time, sit back. lift the tip of the left foot slowly. Repeat the process 7 times.

3) Turning the body to the right and obtaining yin:

Turn the body forward to the right. Push forward slowly with the plams to collect the blue light. Move the body weight forward. Lift the left heel from the ground slowly. While pronouncing " Hong", pull the palms backward slowly, concentrate the mind on conducting the blue light to the lower Dantian along the central vessel. At the same time, sit back. Lift the tip of the right foot slowly. Repeat the process 7 times.

4) Obtaining yin and restoring the primary:

Return to the former standing position. Move and swing the hands downward from the right to the left with the plams facing downward. At the same time, turn the head and body to the right. Switch the body weight to the right, and concentrate the mind on the palms and soles to obtain the blue light from the root of the ground as much as possible. When the two palms reach the same level of the left shouder, they are moving and swinging downward to the right slowly. Simultaneously, turn the head and body to the left. Switch the body weight to the left. While pronouncing "Hong", concentrate the mind on conducting the blue light to the lower Dantian. Obtaining with the left and conducting with the right is considered one process. Repeat the process 7 times. Then, turn the body back to the front, with the two palms drooping at the lateral side of the thighs. "Su Wen. Wu Zang Sheng Cheng Pian" (the Tenth chapter of the Plain Questions) points out:" A person is able to see because there is blood in the liver, able to walk beause there is blood in the feet, able to pinch because there is blood in the fingers" Blood pertains to yin and is marked by quiescence. That is why it is also called "Yin blood", which is the material foundation to nourish and moisten the tissues and zang fu organs of the body, as well as to maintain mental and spiritual activities. Blood deficiency can result in pale complexion, palpitation, poor memory, insomnia, dream disturbed sleeping due to failure of blood nourishment in the heart; dry eyes, weak eye sight due to blood deficiency in the eyes; dry nose and throat, coarse skin and itching, dry stools with hesitant bowel movement due to deficiency of blood in moistening, as well as tremor of the hands and feet, numbness, paralysis of the body and limbs due to failure of blood nourishment in the tendons. Therefore, those who have the above mentioned symptoms of blood deficiency should practise Qigong more. By communicating with the earth, yin blood is tonified, and replenished. All symptoms can be relieved naturally. A person will become stronger and he will be inspired with a high spirit.

Key points to practise this Qigong:

①While obtaining yin and restoring the primary, interlock the movements of the two palms, the head and the body to the left and right which are inter-related. Practise this exercise repeatedly because practice makes perfect.

②Let things take their own course. Yin and yang are different in property. While collecting yang from the heaven, there is a warming sensation running downward from the head; while collecting yin from the earth, there is a cool sensation running upward from the sole; yet, sometimes while collecting heaven yang, there is a cool sensation, and while collecting earth yin, there is a warming sensation, on-the-spot experience is what one has to follow.

③A relative equilibrium of yin and yang should be maintained. The stress in this posture is to collect yin, while the previous one emphasizes collecting yang, yin and yang are inter-dependent. "There exists no solitary yin, nor single yang."

5.Method to refresh the marrow:

Put the two feet together. Hold the ground with the ten toes gently, raise both hands from two sides slowly. Concentrate the mind on obsorbing the white light from the sky and sending it to Laogong (PC 8) and Shixuan (Extra) of the hands. When the palms are above the vertex, infuse the white light to Tian Men. Then put one palm on top of the other. For male, the left hand is below the right; For female, the right hand is below the left.

Leave some space between the two palms, palms and head. Rotate the two palms slowly from the left to right 18 times, taking Tian Men as the centre. Then, rotate the two palms slowly forward to the left from the right 14 times. At the same time, concentrate the mind on the fact that the white light in the sky has penetrated the center of the palm from the dorsal aspect to fill in the head with increasing fullness and brightness. Now, rotate Tian Men, upper, middle and lower Dantian, DiHu, and Eight Diagram of the umbilicus simutaneously and naturally. Relax the whole body. Let qi follow the mind. After rotating clockwise and counter clockwise, put the two palms together, hold Tian Men gently. Close the eyes, watch the interior along the central vessel from Tian Men to the lower Dantian. Finally, move the two palms along the Conception Vessel slowly downward and place them on the umbilicus, concentrate the mind that qi in the whole body converges in the lower Dantian.

This Qigong is called "Methods to refresh the marrow," which obsorbs heavenly yang to refresh both brain marrow and spinal marrow, activates genuine qi running in the central vessel, and disperses in the whole body, enabling spontaneous rotation based on the central vessel. Spontaneous rotation of the Eight Diagram of the Umbilicus promotes the movement and functional activities of the Zangfu organs. The Seventeenth chapter of "Plain Questions" says:"the head is the house of intelligence." Through collecting heavenly yang, brain marrow is refreshed, the circulation of blood vessels in the cranium promoted, and the blood and oxygen supply for cerebral tissues improved. Therefore, this Qigong has its therapeutic effect in healing sequela of cerebro vascular diseases caused by cerebral thrombosis, embolism and hemorrhage, cerebral trauma, sequela of brain concussion, cerebral vascularsclerosis, insufficient blood supply for the brain, headache of various types and intercranial diseases. Moreover, this Qigong is able to regulate the central nervous system in the physiological and biochemical process of the functional activities, regulate the balance between excitation and inhibition of the cerebral cortex, relieve brain diseases caused by atrophy of the cerebral tissues, senile dementia, and menopause syndrome, and neurasthenia, develop the cerebral potential, strengthen the intelligence, the ability of understanding, calculatation, thinking, memorizing, so as to improve the efficacy of study and work, treat alopecia, seborrheic alopeaia, advanced growth of white hair by improving local blood circulation and metabolism of the head.

Key points to practise this Qigong:

1)Hold the ground with the toes gently all the time to obtain essential qi of the root of the earth, and lay a solid foundation to keep the feet strong;

2)Take Tian Men as a centre, rotate the two palms simutaneously;

3)While rotating the two palms clockwise and counter clockwise, concentrate the mind on the white light infusing in the head continuously with brightness;

4)After finishing the practice, conduct qi to the lower Dantian in time because qi should not be retained in the head for long.

6.Method to knock the teeth and generate fluid:

Formula:knock the teeth and stir the saliva with the tongue, blow the cheeks 36 times, swallow the magic saliva by 3 steps to ensure longevity.

Mehtods: Take either a sitting or lying posture. Relax the whole body. Close the eyes gently, calm down and concentrate the mind, be ready to start. Knock the upper teeth with the lower ones 36 times, move the tongue from the left to the right out of the teeth. With the mouth closed, rotate the tongue outside of the upper teeth and lower teeth 9 times clockwise and counter clockwise successively. Blow the cheeks 36 times. The mouth will be full of saliva. (The saliva will be in great amount if one practises more) Then, concentrate the mind on swallowing the saliva to the mouth cavity with audible sound by three steps.

Mechanism and efficacy:

①According to modern scientific tests, saliva created through Qigong practice can increase stomach fluid, which promotes the secretion and digestion of the stomach. Salivary glands are able to compose a kind of hormone which can improve the functions of blood sugar, and be dissolved in blood to regulate the constant of blood sugar with other hormones. So, it is good for all functions of the body.

②The exercise of massage in the mouth cavity with the tongue and by blowing the cheeks can strengthen self-movement of the mouth cavity with preventive effect on the diseases of teeth, throat, and mouth cavity.

③Ancient Chinese people determined the word"活"(live) ("氵"means water;"舌"means tongue) as water on the tongue which means that man lives when there is water on the tongue. A patient at the critical moment, usually has dry lips and tongue. According to Chinese medicine, that is due to failure of ascending of kidney water, resulting in hyperactivity of yang of deficiency type.

This Qigong can generate fluid in the mouth to keep a balance of water and fire, yin and yang. It is effective in treating diseases of hyperactivity of yang due to yin deficiency.

7.Comb the hair and Bathe the face (Sitting or standing posture)

1)Relax the body, close the eyes gently, put the palms together, move the palms to the face. Use two little fingers to press Tian Mu (the midpoint between the two eyebrow). Concentrate the mind on the palms and ten fingers. Raise the head, push gently from Tian Mu along the midline to vertex with slight force of the two little fingers, seperate the other fingers like combing the hair. Bend the head, push further from the vertex to the posterior hair line. Remove the two little fingers after passing through Fengchi (GB 20) bilaterally. Repeat the movement 9 times.

2)Bathe the face: For males, use the left palm first, for female, the right one first. Put the palm transversly on the forehead. Massage from the opposite end of the eyebrow, Sizhukong (TE 23), with slight force of the little finger, passing through supra-orbital bone, forehead, to the supre-orbital bore on the same side, Taiyang (Extra) Ermen (TE 21) Jiache (ST 6) and other points. Then, change the palm, massage from the opposite end of the eyebrow Sizhukong (TE 23) and follow the previous movements. Repeat the whole process 9 times.

Mechanism and efficacy:

This Qigong is able to activate clean yang qi ascending and dispersing all over the head and face, increase the blood circulation and metabolism of the head, enable mental activities to function more logically. So, it has its therapeutic effect in relieving hypertension, cerebral vascular sclerosis, insufficient blood supply for the brain, sequela of C.V.A, dizziness and headache. Meanwhile, it is able to tonify the brain, strengthen the brain, improve the ability of memorizing and thinking. Since the local blood and oxygen supply can be improved, the nutrition struction is renewed, the muscles become tender with luster, white hairs become black, lost hairs regenerated.

8.Method to knead the nose and rub the ear:

1)Method to knead the nose:

Use the middle fingers to knead from Tian Mu, passing the inner canthus, and following the nose bridge on both sides, terminating at Yingxiang (LI 20). Repeat the movement 9 times. Then, press Yingxiang (LI 20) perpendicularly with the tip of the middle finger 9 times, rotate 9 times to the direction of the nostril. Finally, rest the left middle finger at Yingxiang (LI 20) on the left side, knead the right wing of the nose up and down 9 times with the palmar side of the middle finger, rest the right middle finger at Yingxiang (LI 20) on the right side. Knead the left wing of the nose up and down 9 times with the palmar side of the middle finger.

2)Method to rub the root of the ear:

Separate the index and middle fingers of the two hands, hold the root of the ear, rub up and down with light force. Rubbing up and down once is concerned as one movement. Repeat the movement 9 times.

Mechanism and Efficacy:

Through kneading the nose, qi and blood circulation can be promoted, local circulation in the meridians and collaterals can be activated, nose functions of breathing and smelling improved.

So, this Qigong is able to treat both acute and chronic rhinitis, nasal obstruction, loss of sense of smell and distending pain of the forehead. The 28th chapter of "Miraculous Pivot" says: "the ear is the place where all vessels converge." There are corresponding points of the five zang organs and six fu organs, head and face and four limbs inside and outside of the auricle. Rubbing on the ear can not only improve the nourishment of qi and blood of the ear, but also improve the auditory functions, regulate the functions of the zang fu organs, meridians and collaterals of the whole body, play an active role in treating hypertension and various chronic diseases.

9.Method to beat the heavenly drum:

Press the ears tightly with the root of the palms. Be sure qi is not leaking. Tap the occiput 48 times with the left and right fingers alternatively. While tapping, exert finger force slightly and then heavily, slowly and then quickly. Rest the fingers on the occiput and press it. Then, release the root of the palms suddenly. Press tightly again, and release again 3 times. Rotate the posterior part of the ear inside forward and upward with the palmar sides of the fingers. Finally, close the ear orifice with the tips of the index completely. Concentrate the mind on qi being infused to the ear from the tips of the index. After a while, release the tips rapidly with the sound "Bo" to finish the whole process.

Mechanism and Efficacy:

This Qigong was a good method of health preservation in ancient China. It can clear the mind, brighten the eyes, improve the intelligence, and be effective in relieving tinnitis and deafness.

10.Methods to tonify the kidney:

1)Method to rub Yongquan (KI 1)

Hold the left big toe with the left hand, rub gently Yong-quan (KI 1) on the left foot with the right palm at the point Lao gong (PC 8) 81 times (rubbing forward and backward once is one movement). Then change the hand and foot and rub another 81 times.

2)Method to rub Shenshu (BL 23).

Rub the two palms till they are warm. Then rub Shenshu (BL 23) with the palms 81 times.

Mechanism and Efficacy:

Yongquan (KI 1) is a starting point of the kidney meridian. Though Shenshu (BL 23) is a point from the urinary bladder meridian, it is a place where the essential qi of the kidney is stored. Kidney prefers warmth and dislikes cold. The exercise of rubbing the point may tonify and benefit the genuine primary qi of the kidney, strengthen the tendons and bones, be effective in relieving diseases of the genito-urinary system, hyperosteogeny of the lumbar vertebra, knee and low back pain due to kidney deficiency as well as improving reduced vision.

IV.Method of health preservation by diet therapy

1.Cactus Wine

Method of preparation: Select old cactuses which have produced peaches. Scrape off the thorns and coarse peel with a piece of bamboo (any iron-made instrument should not be used). Take 1kg of cactuses and clean them. Put them in an earthen jar, soaked with 1.5 kg pure grain-made wine and 0.5kg crystal sugar, 7 days later, the wine becomes drinkable.

Method of drinking: Drink 5g (of the mine) before each meal, or 5g (of the mine) wherever there is stomachache. The pain will be relieved immediately after drinking it.

Indications: chronic gastritis, stomach ulceration, duodenal ulcer and diseases of digestive system.

precaution: no more than 5g should be taken

each time.

2.Goose Blood

Method of preparation: Take a goose with completely white feathers. Kill it and drink its blood when the blood is still warm. White blood cell count can be increased immediately. Dizziness and palpitation can be relieved at once, immunological functions can be improved. In winter, put a few drops of wine in a bowl, while releasing the blood, stir it with chopsticks to prevent it from freezing. Indications: reduced white blood cell count, dizziness, palpitation, and general lassitude.

3.Rice Porridge with Lotus Seed

Method of preparation: Boil lotus seed with salty water for a while, take off the peel, clean them, and boil them with river or spring water 10 times in an earthenware pot. Then add cleaned rice.

Functions: Calm down the mind, benefit the spleen and stomach, improve hearing and brighten the eyes, moisten the skin and strengthen the health.

4.Rice Porridge with Gorgon Fruit

Method of manufacture: Take off the peels of gorgon fruits first; pound them into pieces. Clean them, and boil them with river or spring water 10 times and then add cleaned rice.

Functions: Gorgon Fruit is sweet in flavour and neutral in property. It pertains to earth, and is not toxic. So, it has the functions in building up the spleen and improving the appetite, relieving low back and knee pain, and tonifying essential qi. It is especially good for aged people. Frequent intake of it is good for health and for prolonging life.

5.Rice Porridge with Milk

Method of manufacture: Soak rice in river water for 24 hours. Then, put it in an enamelled pot with milk from a cattle (or dairy cattle) and boil them 3-5 times. Add prepared rice and boil them together. Thin or thick porridge is made according to the individual taste. Eat it when it is warm.

Indications: Deficiency syndromes of five kinds of strain and seven kinds of impairments.

Functions: Tonify qi and blood, relieve thirst, strengthen the tendons and bones, and prolong life.

6.Method to Eat Longan

Method of eating: Select big longan with green color and rich pulp. Prepare 9 pieces of longan each time to eat at "Zi" "Wu" "Mao" "You" hours(23:00 − 1:00) (11:00 − 13:00) (5:00 − 7:00) (17:00 − 19:00). While eating, sit straightly, facing to either the east or south, getting rid off all disturbing thoughts. Put one piece of longan in the mouth, stir it with the tongue for a while, chew it and remove the kernel, chew the pulp further into paste. At that time, the mouth is full of saliva. So, swallow the pulp paste with saliva by three steps, concentrate the mind that they are sent to the lower Dantian. Eat all the 9 pieces in the same way. This method takes longan as a core where Jing (essence), Qi, Shen (mind) are collected, preserved, and sent to Dantian to perform its warming function, so that "Jing" can be transformed into "qi", and "qi" can be transformed into "Shen". The method of eating longan is also a secret from Taoism, which can strengthen the health and prevent various diseases. There is a saying:"after eating longan, it is miraculous to see that qi returns to its primary source and life is prolonged."

Functions: Nourish the heart and tonify blood, calm down the mind and improve intelligence, relieve palpitation, beautify the complexion, generate essence and prolong life.

7.Tea of Dodder seeds

Method of mannfacture: Dodder seeds, shaped like silkworm seeds live on qi without root. They are collected in autumn and dried in cool place, then cleaned with river water and dried in the sun. Put the seeds in an earthenware pot and roast them with mild fire till they turn yellow. Soak the seeds in boiling water. Drink the water as tea daily.

Functions: Tonify the kidney and strengthen yang, benefit qi and improve strength, tonify marrow and nourish essence.

Indications: weakness, soreness, numbness and pain of the low back and knees with difficulty in walking, weakness of the four limbs, nocturnal emission, etc. Frequent drinking of this tea strengthens the tendons and bones, brighten the eyes and prolongs life.

8.Tea of Flattened milkvetch seed

Method of manufacture: Flattened milkvetch seed is nontoxic, sweet and pungent in flavour, warm in property. It has two colors, white and black. The one with black color is a granule and in the form of the kidney. It is mostly produced in Sha yuan (Henan province). That is why it is called shayuan jili. The two types have the same functions. If the seeds are white in color, roast them into deep-yellow color in an earthenware pot. Remove the thorns with stone instruments. Clean and dry them in a cool place. If the seeds are black, chean them with water, and dry them in the sun, then roast them with mild fire till they smell good.

Functions: Tonify the kidney, brighten the eyes, resolve tumors and masses.

Indications: discharge of leukorrhea, laryngitis, hemorrhoid complicated by anal fistula.

This tea ensures a relexed body with good health and long life.

9.Rice Porridge with Chinese Yam

Method of manufacture: Chinese Yam is collected in autumn and dried in the sun. Pound and sieve it into a powder. Cook it with rice and eat both.

Functions and indications: Chinese Yam is non-toxic, sweet in flavour, warm and neutral in property. It acts on Taiyin meridians of the hand and foot, and tonifies the spleen and stomach, moistens the skin, and strengthens the tendons and bones, relieves restlessness and severe, intermittant headache.

10.Pills of genuine Yang

Method of manufacture: Use some fresh deer horns, (the dosage is not specifically mentioned) make them into powder and mix with qualified wine and dry them, mix with wine again. Repeat this process 9 times, then roast them till they are deep-yellow, but not burned, with a mild fire. Grind them into a fine powder. Mix the powder evenly with prepared white honey. Make them into pills (as big as the seeds of a Chinese parasol tree) Dry them a bit, and sotre them in an enamelled container for use. Eat 3g every morning and evening with light salty water.

Functions: The pills are efficacious medicine for health preservation and longevity with the functions of tonifying the kidney and controlling essence, improving hearing and brightening the eyes.

Indications: poor memory, severe palpitation, weakness of the low back and knees, weakness of the four limbs, various diseases caused by qi and blood deficiency.

Remarks on Viewing Taiji Diagram
(in the begining of the book)

Taiji Diagram is a symbol, revealing the changes of the universe. Having assumed a posture for Qigong practice, the Qigong practitioner looks once at the diagram, then closes his eyes with the

Taiji Diagram at Dantian(Elixir Field)for the purpose of increasing the Qi sensation and the efficacy of Qigong practice.

When the practitioner is a patient, he should look for a while at the diagram and close his eyes with the image of the diagram at the affected region of his disease, or at a painful site: this conduction serves to remove Qi and blood stagnation,smooth the flow of qi and dredge the meridians and collaterals in order to eliminate the disease and strengthen the body resistance.

VI.The Mechanism of Magnetic Apparatus in Healing Diseases

The human body is a mild electric field, a magnetic field, emitting infra red light. These constitute the biological field. The physiological and pathological state of the human body can be reflected in currently used common medical instruments through the changed electric field and magnetic field of the body.With the help of the instruments, diagnosis can be made.

The activity of the biological field of a healthy person is vigorous, whereas, its activity in a weak person is feeble.

Qigong therapy enhances the orderliness and synchronization of the electric current and the magnetic field of muscles, nerves and organs by regulating the electric field and the magnetic field of various parts of the human body. The balance of the electric field and the magnetic field of the body harmed either by external causes, such as trauma, bacteria, viruses, excessive physical exertion, or internal factors, like moodiness, for instance, which cause malaise or illnesses. Each part of the human body and its tissues and cells contain an electric field. The part or tissue generating an electric field also has a corresponding magnetic field. Disturbance of the electric and magnetic fields gives rise to the onset of diseases.

The human body is a great electric field, coexisting with the magnetic field. There are cerebral electric magnetic field, the cardiac electric magnetic field, the other external and internal organs' electric magnetic fields, and the muscular electric magnetic field. These fields not only influence each other, but also spread their influence all over the body. The phenomenon exhibits that malaise in a certain part of the body is often associated with the malaise of other parts of the body. The occurrence of a disease frequently complicates other diseases.

When the electric field of the human body is reinforced, the emission of infra – red light and microwaves is also reinforced. When a person is in a Qigong state, a warm sensation or a tingling sensation may be felt in some parts of the body and in some organs. In addition, attraction or rebelling between some acupoints as well as light, flying feelings are also perceived. These phenomena are the perception of the reinforcement of a person's own biological field. The reinforced biological field not only plays a special role in the cellular metabolism, proliferation and functioning, but also exerts strong inhibition and the destruction of bacteria and destroys cells. As the electro magnetic field dilates the capillaries, strengthens the activity of enzymes, promotes cellular metabolism, increases the volume of the white blood cells and enhances phagocytosis, Qigong practice is, therefore, the process of self reinforcement of the biological field, the process of healing illness, and keeping fit.

The currently available magnetic apparatus are the supplementary instruments for health preservation purposes. Their preventive and curative mechanism derives from the fact that the human body is an electro magnetic field.

Heaven and earth contain magnetic fields, the magnetic field of nature exerts its influence on the magnetic field of the hunan body. The aim of Qigong practice is to coordinate with the natural magnetic field, and to keep the individual's magnetic field in a balanced state. When the human body undergoes certain imbalances and a disease occurs, physical and chemical approaches, such as medication and medical instruments are resorted to in order to stimulate certain organs to regain the balance of the magnetic field. Thus healing the affected or weakened tissues, and the purpose of restoring health is achieved.

The Ba Gua Brand Keeping Fit Magnetic Couple Balls introduced herein is a third generation product, developed from the traditional Chinese health keeping balls. They are designed on the basis of magnetic therapy, integrating the doctrine of Chinese medicine which holds that the ten fingers communicate with the heart. Through the action of the magnetic field, the fingers through the arms connect with the central nervous system, the viscera and the blood vessels. In the exercise the magnetic balls are rotated in the palms, stimulating the acupoints located in the center of the palms, the dorsum of hands and fingers, and keeping a smooth flow of Qi and bood in the meridians and collaterals. The exercise with the magnetic balls has a good effect on the inflammation of nerve endings, numbness and contracture of the hands and arms, hemiplegia, arthritis, hypertension and tumors, and is particularly good for the weak and for senile patients. Introduction of the keeping fit magnetic couple balls is aimed at providng patients or Qigong practitioners, whose Qigong efficacy is not high, with a supplementary way of stimulating the relevant acupoints for self preservation of health. To avoid some possible problems, other magnetic apparatus are not recommended here as their properties and effects are unknown to the author. The keeping fit magnetic couple balls which are patented are solely manufactured by Xiaba Health Preservation Products Manufacturer.

VII. Methods of Using Keeping Fit Magnetic Couple Balls

1. Turn the ball in the palm with fingers. It can be done in one hand, for workers who use mental energy it is better to use the left hand, or both hands for promoting brain function and intelligence.

2. Assume the sitting or lying posture with one or two balls under the soles of the feet (preferably in bare feet); press the balls under the sole in a back and forth movement or rotating movement in order to stimulate Yongquan (KI 1), to promote brain function. For children under the age of 15, this method promotes healthy growth and intelligence and is significant in increasing height.

3. If the user is a patient,he should put the attraction point of the ball displayed when two balls are attracted, on a relevant acupoint (most acupoints are symmetrically located) or a painful site, massaging the point with the ball in an up and down motion or in clockwise rotation. If the

patient can not apply the massage himself he can be helped by others. The massage is performed for over 20 min. and applied 2-3 times daily.

4. Lay the attraction point of the ball on the side opposite to the affected site or an acupoint to cause the magnetic line go through the point. This will enhance the curative effect.

5. Wash the magnetic ball to clean it. Put the ball into cold water, stir the ball around for 1 minute, then take the ball out of the water. The water thus becomes magnetized and can be drunk after being boiled. If one drinks the magnetized water frequently,the urinary system stones, hypertension, diabetes, and enterogastric disorders can be treated, or the health of a person without disease will be reinforced.

Precautions for Using the Magnetic Balls

1. If the phenomena of palpitations, dizziness, etc., which may occur among a few users, appear, stop applying the therapy. There is no need to perform any special management.

2. Be careful not to knock the ball or lay it on an overly hot place. If the balls collide accidently, shaking the parts inside the balls, the magnetic force should not decrease. In general, the therapeutic effect will not be influenced.

3. Lay the balls far away from clocks, wrist watches, TV and tape recorder so as to avoid magnetization.

4. The balls can be used for over 5 years.

The Ba Gua Brand magnetic ball product has attained a patent. The patent is No.2411. It is produced solely by Xiaba Health Preservation product Manufacturer.

CHAPTER 2

Ⅰ. METHODS OF LOCATING POINTS

Finger measurement is one of the commonly used methods of locating acupoints. The length and width of the patient's finger(s) are taken as a standard for point location. The following four methods are presented:

1.Middle finger measurement

The length of the second interphalangeal joint of the middle finger is taken as one cun.

2.Thumb measurement

The width of the interphalangeal joint of the thumb is taken as one cun.

3.Two-finger measurement

The width of the closed index and middle fingers is taken as one and half cun.

4.Four-finger measurement

The width of the closed index, middle, ring and little fingers is taken as three cun.

II.POINTS FOR THE COMMON DISEASES AND THEIR LOCATIONS

1.Headache

Yintang (Ex-HN 3),Baihui (GV 20), NaoHu (GV 17), Tianzhu (BL 10), Yuzhen(BL 9), Toulinqi(GB 15), Houding (GV 19), Hegu(LI 4), Kunlun (BL 60), Fengfu (GV 16),Muchuang (GB 16), Taichong (LR 3), Yangbai (GB 14), Chengguang (BL 6), Guanchong (TE 1), Fenglong (ST 40), Qingling (HT 2), Zhongzhu (TE 3), Taiyang (Ex-HN 5).

1) Yintang (Ex-HN3)

Location: Midway between the medial ends of the two eyebrows.

Function: To expel wind, promote resusciation, clear away heat and remove toxin.

2) Baihui (GV 20)

Location: On the centre of the head, 5 cun posterior to the anterior hairline and 7 cun anterior to the posterior hairline.

Function: To clear away heat, open the orifice,

rescue yang from the collapse, pacify the liver yang and calm down the mind.

3) Naohu (GV 17)

Location: Superior to the external occipital protuberance, 1.5 cun directly above Fengfu (GV 16).

Function: To promote resusciation, stop pain and tranquilize the mind.

4) Tianzhu (BL 10)

Location: 1.3 cun lateral to Yamen (GV 15), on the lateral aspect of m. trapezius.

Function: To relieve dizziness and open the orifice.

5) Yuzhen (BL 9)

Location: On the lateral side of the superior border of the external occipital protuberance, 1 cun posterior to Luoque (BL 8) and 1.3 cun lateral to Naohu (GV 17).

Function: To relieve pain and calm down the mind.

6) Toulinqi (GV 15)

Location: Eyes are stared forward, 0.5 cun within the hairline, directly above the puples, midway between Shenting (GV 24) and Touwei (ST 8).

Function: To calm down the mind and promote

circulation in the meridian and collateral.

7) Houding (GV 19)

Location: On the back of the head, 1.5 cun directly above Qiangjian (GV18).

Function: To clear away heat and relieve pain.

8) Hegu (LI 4)

Location: On the dorsum of the hand, in the depression between the 1st and 2nd metacarpal bones.

Function: To expel wind, eliminate the exterior syndormes, promote qi and blood circulation in the meridian and collateral, open the orifice and stop pain.

9) Kunlun (BL 60)

Location: In the depression posterior to the external malleolus.

Function: To expel wind, promote circulation in the collateral, relax tendons, strengthen the lumbus and calm down the mind.

10) Fengfu (GV 16)

Location: Directly below the occipital protuberance, in the depression between m. trapezius of both sides.

Function: To dispel wind and eliminate the pathogenic factors.

11) Muchuang (GB 16)

Location: Eyes are stared forward, directly above the pupil, two cun within the hairline, 1.5 cun posterior to Toulinqi (GB 15), on the line connecting Toulinqi (GB 15) and Fengchi (GB 20).

Function: To expel wind and disperse heat, clear the mind and brighten the eyes.

12) Taichong (LR 3)

Location: On the dorsum of the foot, in the depression distal to the junction of the 1st and 2nd metatarsal bones.

Function: To pacify the liver qi, activate the circulation of blood and remove stagnation.

13) Yangbai (GB 14)

Location: Eyes are stared forward, directly above the pupil, one cun above the midpoint of the eyebrow. On the connecting point of the upper 2/3 and the lower 1/3 of the line between the anterior hairline and the eyebrow.

Function: To expel wind and stop pain.

14) Chengguang (BL 6)

Location: On the head, 1.5 cun posterior to Wuchu (BL 5).

Function: To open the orifice and calm down the mind.

15) Guanchong (TE 1)

Location: On the lateral side of the ring finger,

about 0.1 cun posterior to the corner of the nail.

Function: To clear away fire from the Triple Energizers, relieve heat and stop pain.

16) Fenglong (ST 40)

Location: 8 cun anterior and superior to the external malleolus, the midway between the low border of patella and the midpoint of the external malleolus.

Function: To clear the mind, promote the circulation of qi and ascend yang.

17) Qingling (HT 2)

Location: On the medial aspect of the elbow, 3 cun above Shaohai (HT 3).

Function: To promote circulation in the meridian and collateral.

18) Zhongzhu (TE 3)

Location: On the dorsum of the hand between the 4th and 5th metacarpal bones, in the depression proximal to the metacarpophalangeal joint.

Function: To open the orifice, benefit the brain, expel wind and clear away heat.

19) Taiyang (Ex-HN 5)

Location: In the depression about 1 cun posterior to the midpoint between the lateral end of the eyebrow and the outer canthus.

Function: To disperse wind, clear away heat,

brighten the eyes and open the orifice.

2.Migraine

Taiyang (Ex-HN 5), Fengchi (GB 20), Zheng-ying (GB 17), Tianjing (TE 10), Touwei (ST 10), Sizhukong (TE 23),Yangfu (GB 38), Zuqiaoyin (GB 44), Sidu (TE 9), Jianjing (GB 21), Shuaigu (GB 8), Xuanzhong (GB 39).

1) Taiyang (Ex-HN5)

Location: In the depression about 1 cun posterior to the midpoint between the lateral end of the eyebrow and the outer canthus.

Function: To disperse wind, eliminate heat, brighten the eyes and open the orifice.

2) Fengchi (GB 20)

Location: In the depression between the upper portion of m. sternocleidomastoideus and m. trape-zius, below the occipital bone.

Function: To disperse wind, eliminate heat, promote circulation in the meridian and collateral, brighten the eyes and open the orifice.

3) Zhengying (GB 17)

Location: 1.5 cun posterior to Muchuang (GB 16), on the line joining Toulingqi (GB 15) and Fengchi (GB 20).

Function: To disperse wind, clear away heat, brighten the eyes and open the orifice.

4) Tianjing (TE 10)

Location: In the depression between two tendons, posterior to the major bone on the lateral aspect of the elbow, about 1 cun posterior and superior to the olecranon of the ulna.

Function: To brighten the eyes, benefit the brain and lubricate joints.

5) Touwei (ST 8)

Location: Directly above the centre between the medial ends of two eyebrows, 0.5 cun within the hairline and 4.5 cun lateral to the midline of the forehead.

Function: To clear away heat and stop pain.

6) Sizhukong (TE 23)

Location: In the depression at the lateral end of the eyebrow.

Function: To disperse wind, clear away heat, open the orifice and benefit the brain.

7) Yangfu (GB 38)

Location: 4 cun above the external malleolus, on the anterior border of the fibula.

Function: To promote circulation in the meridian and collateral, disperse wind and eliminate damp.

8) Zuqiaoyin (GB 44)

Location: On the lateral side of the fourth toe,

about 0.1 cun posterior to the corner of the nail.

Function: To descend qi and clear away fire from the Upper Energizer.

9) Sidu (TE 9)

Location: On the lateral aspect of the forearm, 5 cun below the elbow, on the anterior border of the ulna.

Function: To disperse wind, stop pain and promote circulation in the meridian and collateral.

10) Jianjing (GB 21)

Location: Midway between Dazhu (CV 14) and the acromion.

Function: To promote circulation in the meridian and collateral, expel wind, stop pain, relax the chest and descend the upward perversion of qi.

11) Shuaigu (GB 8)

Location: Superior to the apex of the auricle, 1.5 cun within the hairline.

Function: To promote circulation in the meridian and collateral, disperse wind and open the orifice.

12) Xuanzhong (GB 39)

Location: 3 cun above the tip of the external malleolus, slightly anterior to the fibula.

Function: To promote circulation in the meridiar and collateal, disperse wind and eliminate damp.

3. Dizziness

Taichong (LR 3), Baihui (GV 20), Tongtian (BL 7), Tongli (HT 5), Xinhui (GV 22), Shenzhu (GV 12), Shenmai (BL 62), Sibai (ST 2), Renzhong (GV 26), Tianzhu (BL 10), Zhongchong (PC 9), Muchuang (GB 16), Yintang (Ex-HN3), Shenting (GV 24), Naohu (GV 17), Taodao (GV 13), Yongquan (KI 1).

1) Taichong (LR 3)

Location: On the dorsum of the foot, in the depression distal to the junction of the 1st and 2nd metatarsal bones.

Function: To pacify the liver qi, activate the circulation of blood and remove stagnation.

2) Baihui (GV 20)

Location: On the centre of the vertax, 5 cun posterior to the anterior hairline and 7 cun anterior to the posterior hairline.

Function: To clear away heat, open the orifice, rescue yang from the collapse, pacify the liver qi, disperse wind and calm down the mind.

3) Tongtian (BL 7)

Location: 1.5 cun posterior to Chengguan (BL 6) on the head.

Funciton: To promote the circulation of qi in the meridian, open the upper orifice so as to conduct qi to the vertax, Baihui (GV 20), along the distribution of the meridian of Foot-Taiyang.

4) Tongli (HT 5)

Location: On the radial side of the tendon of m. flexor carpi ulnaris, 1 cun above the transverse crease of the wrist.

Function: To promote circulation in the meridian and collateral, calm down the mind and tranquilize the mind.

5) Xinhui (GV 22)

Location: 2 cun posterior to the anterior hairline, 3 cun anterior to Baihui (GV 20).

Function: To build up the spirits, stop pain and tranquilize the mind.

6) Shenzhu (GV 12)

Location: Below the spinous process of the third thoracic vertebra.

Function: To strengthen the antipathogenic qi.

7) Shenmai (BL 62)

Location: In the depression, 0.5 cun below the inferior border of the external malleolus.

Function: To calm down the mind, ralex tendons and promote circulation in the meridion.

8) Sibai (ST 2)

Location: To stare forward, directly below the pupil, in the depression at the infraorbital foramen.

Function: To clear away heat and disperse wind.

9) Renzhong (Shuigou) (GV 26)

Location: Below the nose, on the midline of the philtrum, at the junction between the upper 1/3 and lower 2/3.

Function: To clear away heat, open the orifice, calm down the mind, regain yang from the collapse. It is the emergent point for all cases of loss of consciousness.

10) Tianzhu (BL 10)

Location: 1.3 cun lateral to Yamen (GV 15), on the lateral aspect of m. trapezius.

Function: To clear the mind and open the orifice.

11) Zhengchong (PC 9)

Location: In the centre of the tip of the middle finger.

Function: To rescue yang from the collapse, open the orifice, and promote circulation in the meridian. It is one of the key points for the emergency.

12) Muchuang (GB 16)

Location: To stare forward, directly above the pupil, 2 cun within the hairline, on the connecting line between Toulinqi (GB 15) and Fengchi (GB 20).

Function: To dispel wind, eliminate heat, clear the mind and brighten the eyes.

13) Yintang (Ex-HN 3)

Location: On the forehead, in the centre between the two medial ends of the eyebrows.

Function: To disperse wind, clear the mind, clear away heat and remove toxin.

14) Shenting (GV 24)

Location: 0.5 cun directly above the midpoint of the anterior hairline.

Function: To rescue yang from the collapse.

15) Naohu (GV 17)

Location: 1.5 cun directly above Fengfu (GV 16), superior to the external occipital protuberance.

Function: To clear the mind, stop pain and tranquilize the mind.

16) Taodao (GV 13)

Location: Below the spinous process of the first thoracic vertebra.

Function: To clear away heat and expel wind.

17) Yongquan (KI 1)

Location: On the sole, in the depression when the foot is in plantar flexion.

Function: To promote circulation in the meridian and collateral, nourish yin, reduce fire, nourish the liver to eliminate wind, open the orifice and calm down the mind.

4.Trigeminal Neuralgia

Xiaguan(ST 7), Taiyang (Ex-HN5), Wangu (SI 4), Yangbai (GB 14), Zanzhu (BL 2),Quanliao (SI 18).

1) Xiaguan (ST 7)

Location: In the depression formed by the zygomatic arch and the mandibular notch.

Function: To clear away heat and stop pain.

2) Taiyang (Ex-HN5)

Location: In the depression about 1 cun posterior to the midpoint between the lateral end of the eyebrow and the outer canthus.

Function: To expel wind, eliminate heat, brighten the eyes and open the orifice.

3) Wangu (SI 4)

Location: The fist is made, on the junction of the white and red skin, between the base of the fifth metacarpal bone and the triquetral bone.

Function: To disperse wind and promote circulation in the meridian and collateral.

4) Yangbai (GB 14)

Location: To stare forward, directly above the pupil, one cun directly above the midpoint of the eyebrow, at the junction of the upper 2/3 and lower 1/3 of the line connecting the anterior hairline and the eyebrow.

Function: To expel wind and relieve pain.

5) Zanzhu (BL 2)

Location: In the depression on the medial extremity of the eyebrow, above Jingming (BL 1).

Function: To disperse wind, brighten the eyes, clear the mind and stop pain.

6) Quanliao (SI 18)

Location: Dirctly below the outer canthus, in the depression on the lower border of zygoma.

Function: To expel wind, clear away heat and promote circulation of the meridian and collateral.

5. Facial Paralysis

Renzhong (GV 26), Taiyang (Ex-HN5), Fengchi (GB 20), Xiaguan (ST 7), Sibai (ST 2), Sizhukong (TE 23), Dicang (ST 4), Yifeng (TE 17), Tongziliao (GB 1), Hegu (LI 4), Xingjian (LR 2), Chongyang (ST 42),Yingxiang (LI 20), Chengjiang (CV 24).

1) Renzhong (GV 26) (Shuigou)

Location: Below the nose, on the junction of the upper 1/3 and lower 2/3 of the philtrum.

Function: To clear away heat, open the orifice calm down the mind and rescue yang from the collapse. It is the emergent point for all cases of loss of consciousness.

2) Taiyang (Ex-HN5)

Location: In the depression about 1 cun posterior to the midpoint between the lateral end of the eyebrow and the outer canthus.

Function: To disperse wind, clear away heat, brighten the eyes and open the orifice.

3) Fengchi (GB 20)

Location: In the depression between the upper portion of m. sternocleidomastoideus and m. trapezius.

Function: To disperse wind, eliminate heat, promote circulation in the meridian and collateral, brighten the eyes and open the orifice.

4) Xiaguan (ST 7)

Location: In the depression formed by the zygomatic arch and the mandibular notch.

Function: To clear away heat and stop pain.

5) Sibai (ST 2)

Location: To stare forward, directly below the pupil, in the depression at the infraorbital foramen.

Function: To clear away heat and disperse wind.

6) Sizhukong (TE 23)

Location: In the depression at the lateral end of the eyebrow.

Function: To expel wind, clear away heat, open the orifice and benefit the brain.

7) Dicang (ST 4)

Location: 0.4 cun lateral to the corner of the mouth, in m. orbicularis oris.

Function: To eliminate pathogenic wind, clear the mind and tranquilize the mind.

8) Yifeng (TE 17)

Location: Posterior to the lobule of the ear, between the mandible and mastoid process, in the depression when the mouth is opened.

Function: To expel wind, promote circulation in the meridian and collateral, open the orifice and benefit the brain.

9) Tongziliao (GB 1)

Location: 0.5 cun lateral to the outer canthus, on the lateral aspect of the orbit.

Function: To disperse wind, eliminate heat, clear the mind and brighten the eyes.

10) Hegu(LI 4)

Location: In the depression between the 1st and 2nd metacarpal bones, on the dorsum of the hand.

Function: To expel wind, eliminate the exterior syndromes, promote the circulation of qi and blood in the meridian, open the orifice and stop pain.

11) Xingjian (LR 2)

Location:Between the 1st and 2nd toes, 0.5 cun

posterior to the margin of the web.

Function: To promote circulation in the meridian and collateral and pacify the liver yang.

12) Chongyang (ST 42)

Location: In the depression among the 2nd and 3rd metatarsal bones and the cuneiform bone, 1.5 cun directly below Jiexi (ST 41)

Function: To activate the blood circulation in the meridian, harmonize the stomach functions and stop pain.

13) Yingxiang (LI 20)

Location: Between the nasolabial groove and the midpoint of the lateral border of ala nasi.

Function: To remove nasal obstruction and treat facial paralysis.

14) Chengjiang (CV 24)

Location: On the midline of the lower jaw, superior to the border of the lower lip, in the depression of the centre of the mentolabial groove.

Function: To expel wind, promote circulation in the meridion and stop pain.

6. Neurasthenia, Insomnia

Xinshu (BL15), Shenmen (HT 7), Lidui (ST 45), Zhongwan (CV 12), Shenting (GV 24), Gaohuang-shu (BL 43), Zusanli (ST 36), Zulinqi (GB 41), Zuqiaoyin (GB 44), Zhaohai (KI 6), Yongquan (KI

1) Xinshu (BL 15)

Location: 1.5 cun lateral to the lower border of the spinous process of the 5th thoracic vertebra.

Function: To tranquilize the mind.

2) Shenmen (HT 7)

Location: In the depression on the ulnar aspect of the transverse crease of the wrist. To locate the point avoiding to the artery.

Function: To calm down the mind and promote circulation in the meridian.

3) Lidu (ST 45)

Location: Between the 2nd and 3rd toes, in the depression anterior and lateral to the 2nd meta-tarsodigital joint.

Function: To tranquilize the mind.

4) Zhongwan (CV 12)

Location: On the midline of the abdomen, 4 cun above the umbilicus.

Function: To descend the upward perversion of qi, eliminate mild heat, regulate the circulation of qi and harmonize the stomach functions.

5) Shenting (GV 24)

Location: 0.5 cun directly above the midpoint of the anterior hairline.

Function: To rescue yang from the collapse.

6) Gaohuangshu (BL 43)

Location: 3 cun lateral to the lower border of the spinous process of the fourth thoracic vertabra.

Function: To calm down the mind, benefit the brain, and rescue yang from the collapse.

7) Zusanli (ST 36)

Location: 3 cun below the patella, one finger-breadth from the anterior crest of the tibia.

Function: To calm down the mind, stop pain and tonify qi and blood.

8) Zulinqi (GB 41)

Location: In the depression anterior to the junction of the 4th and 5th metatarsal bones.

Function: To calm down the mind, pacify the liver qi and brighten the eyes.

9) Zuqiaoyin (GB 44)

Location: On the lateral side of the 4th toe, about 0.5 cun posterior to the corner of the nail.

Function: To conduct qi flowing downward and clear away fire from the Upper Energizer.

10) Zhaohai (KI 6)

Location: In the depression directly below the medial malleolus.

Function: To calm down the mind, activate the circulation of blood and relieve pain.

11) Yongquan (KI 1)

Location: On the sole, in the depression when the foot is in plantar flexion.

Function: To promote circulation in the meridian and collateral, nourish yin to reduce fire, nourish the liver functions to reduce wind, open the orifice and clam down the mind.

7. Epilepsy

Renzhong (GV 26), Shangwan (CV 13), Xiaohai (SI 8), Zhizheng (SI 7), Tianzhu (BL 10), Fenglong (ST 40), Taiyi (ST 23), Juque (CV 14), Shaochong (HT 9), Fengfu (GV 16), Xinshu (BL 15), Shenmai (BL 62), Baihui (GV 20), Houxi (SI 3), Shenzhu (GV 12), Jianshi (PC 5), Chengguang (BL 6), Shenting (GV 24), Naohu (GV 17), Yongquan (KI 1), Zhubin (KI 9), Zhaohai (KI 6), Jiuwei (CV 15) which is applied when epilepsy attacks during the night.

1) Renzhong (GV 26) (Shuigou)

Location: On the junction of the upper 1/3 and lower 2/3 of the midline of the philtrum.

Function: To clear away heat, regain consciousness, open the orifice, calm down the mind, rescue yang from the collapse. It is the emergent point for all cases of loss of consciousness.

2) Shangwan (CV 13)

Location: On the midline of the abdomen, 5 cun above the umbilicus.

Function: To regulate the circulation of qi.

3) Xiaohai (SI 8)

Location: When the elbow is flexed, the point is located in the depression between the olecranon of the ulna and the medial epicondyle of the humerus.

Function: To expel wind and promote circulation in the meridian.

4) Zhizheng (SI 7)

Location: On the line joining Yanggu (SI 5) and Xiaohai (SI 8), 5 cun posterior to the wrist.

Function: To promote circulation in the meridian and collateral, expel wind and clear away heat.

5) Tianzhu (BL 10)

Location: 1.3 cun lateral to Yamen (GV 15), on the lateral aspect of m. trapezius.

Function: To open the orifice and remove dizziness.

6) Fenglong (ST 40)

Location: 8 cun anterior and superior to the external malleolus, the midpoint between the lower border of the patella and the external malleolus.

Fouction: To clear the mind, smooth the circulation of qi and elevate yang.

7) Taiyi (ST 23)

Location: 2 cun above the umbilicus and 2 cun lateral to the midline of the abdomen.

Function: To tranquilize the mind and relieve pain.

8) Juque (CV 14)

Location: On the midline of the abdomen, 6 cun above the umbilicus.

Function: To descend the upward perversion of qi of Zang organs.

9) Shaochong (HT 9)

Location:On the radial side of the little finger, about 0.1 cun posterior to the corner of the nail.

Function: To regulate the circulation of qi in the meridian and tranquilize the mind.

10) Fengfu (GV 16)

Location: Directly below the external occipital protuberance, in the depression between m. trapezius of both sides, on the most upper region of the vertebral joint.

Function: To expel wind and eliminate pathogenic factors.

11) Xinshu (BL 15)

Location: 1.5 cun lateral to the lower border of the spinous process of the fifth thoracic vertebra.

Function: To tranquilize the mind.

12) Shenmai (BL 62)

Location: In the depression, 0.5 cun below the external malleolus.

Function: To relax tendons, promote circulation in the meridian, and tranquilize the mind.

13) Baihui (GV 20)

Location: In the centre of the vertax, 5 cun posterior to the anterior hairline and 7 cun anterior to the posterior hairline.

Function: To relieve heat, open the orifice, rescue yang from the collapse, pacify the liver wind and tranquilize the mind.

14) Houxi (SI 3)

Location: When a loose fist is made, the point is on the ulnar side, proximal to the fifth metacarpophalangeal joint, at the end of the transverse crease.

Function: To clear away heat, expel wind, promote circulation in the meridian and collateral.

15) Shenzhu (GV 12)

Location: Below the spinous process of the third thoracic vertebra.

Function: To strengthen the antipathogenic qi.

16) Jianshi (PC 5)

Location: 3 cun above the transverse crease of the wrist, on the flexion aspect of the forearm, between the tendons of m. palmaris longus and m.

flexor carpi radialis.

Function: To calm down the mind and promote circulation in the meridian and collateral.

17) Chengguang (BL 6)

Location: 1.5 cun posterior to Wuchu (BL 5), on the vertax.

Function: To open the orifice and calm down the mind.

18) Shenting (GV 24)

Location 0.5 cun directly above the midpoint of the anterior hairline.

Function: To rescue yang from the collapse.

19) Naohu (GV 17)

Location: 1.5 cun directly above Fengfu (GV 16),superior to the external occipital protuberance.

Function: To build up the spirits, stop pain and tranquilize the mind.

20) Yongquan (KI 1)

Location On the sole, in the depression when the foot is in plantar flexion.

Function: To promote circulation in the meridian and collateral, nourish yin to reduce fire, nourish the liver functions to pacify wind, open the orifice and tranquilize the mind.

21) Zhubin (KI 9)

Location: 5 cun directly above Taixi (KI 3) at

the lower end of the belly of m. gastrocnemius.

Function: To calm down the mind, disperse wind and regulate the circulation of qi.

22) Zhaohai (KI 6)

Location:In the depression, 1 cun directly below the medial malleolus.

Function: To activate the circulation of blood, relieve pain, and tranquilize the mind.

23) Jiuwei (CV 15)

Location: Below the xiphoid process, 7 cun above the umbilicus; to locate the point in the supine position with the arms uplifted and holding the head.

Function: To calm down the mind, regulate the circulation of qi and stop pain. The point is commonly applied when epilepsy attacks during the night.

8. Toothache

Yinjiao (GV 28), Touwei(ST 8), Sanyangluo (TE 8),Xiaguan (ST 7), Juliao (ST 3), Neiting (ST 44), Zhengying (GB 17), Sidu (TE 9), Waiguan (TE 5), Sizhukong (TE 23), Hegu (LI 4), Chengjiang (CV 24), Shangyang (LI 1), Jiache (ST 6), Quanliao (SI 18).

1) Yinjiao (GV 28)

Location: At the junction of the gum and the

frenulum of the upper lip.

Function: To connect Governor and Conception vessels.

2) Touwei (ST 8)

Location: 0.5 cun directly above the midpoint of the anterior hairline and about 4.5 cun lateral to the midline of the forehead.

Function: To clear away heat and stop pain.

3) Sanyangluo (TE 8)

Location: 4 cun posterior to the transverse crease of the dorsum of the wrist, between the radius and ulna.

Function: To disperse wind, clear away heat, open the orifice and benefit the brain.

4) Xiaguan (ST 7)

Location: In the depression formed by the anterior zygomatic arch and mandibular notch.

Function: To clear away heat and stop pain.

5) Juliao (ST 3)

Location: To stare forward, directly below the pupil, at the level with the lower border of ala nasi.

Function: To expel wind and promote circulation in the meridian.

6) Neiting (ST 44)

Location: In the depression, about 0.5 cun

posterior to the web margin between the 2nd and 3 rd toes, on the dorsum of the foot.

Function: To regulate the circulation of qi and stop pain.

7) Zhengying (GB 17)

Location: 1.5 cun posterior to Muchuang (GB 16), on the line joining Toulinqi (GB 15) and Fengchi (GB 20).

Function: To disperse wind, clear away heat, brighten the eyes and open the orifice.

8) Sidu (TE 9)

Location: On the dorsal aspect of the forearm, 5 cun below the elbow, on the anterior border of the ulna.

Function: To disperse wind, stop pain and promote circulation in the meridian and collateral.

9) Waiguan (TE 5)

Location: 2 cun posterior to the transverse crease of the wirst, between the radius and ulna, on the dorsal aspect of the forearm.

Function: To disperse the exterior syndromes, clear away heat and promote circulation in the meridian and collateral.

10) Sizhukong (TE 23)

Location: In the depression at the lateral end of the eyebrow.

Function: To disperse wind, clear away heat, open the orifice and benefit the brain.

11) Hegu (LI 4)

Location: On the dorsum of the head, in the depression between the 1st and 2nd metacarpal bones.

Function: To disperse wind, eliminate the exterior syndromes, promote the circulation of qi and blood in the meridian, open the orifice, and stop pain.

12) Chengjiang (CV 24)

Location: On the midline of the mandible superior to the border of the lower lip, in the depression of the centre of the mentolabial groove.

Function: To disperse wind, promote circulation in the meridian to relieve pain and stop spasm.

13) Shangyang (LI 1)

Location: On the radial side of the index finger, about 0.1 cun posterior to the corner of the nail.

Function: To clear away heat and ease pain.

14) Jiache (ST 6)

Location: On m. masseter, anterior and superior to the lower angle of the mandible, on the prominence of the muscle when the teeth clenched or in the depression when the mouth is opened.

Function: To relieve swelling and eliminate the pathogenic factors.

15) Quanliao (SI 18)

Location: Dirctly below the outer canthus, in the depression on the lower border of zygoma.

Function: To disperse wind, clear away heat and promote circulation in the meridian and collateral.

9. Periarthritis of Shoulder

Dazhu(BL 11), Shanglian (LI 9), Jugu (LI 16), Shousanli (LI 10), Quyuan (SI 13), Tiaokou (ST 38), Bingfeng (SI 12), Jianjing (GB 21), Jianzhen (SI 9), Jianyu (LI 15).

1) Dazhu (BL 11)

Location: 1.5 cun lateral to the lower border of the spinous process of the 1st thoracic vertebra, about two-finger width lateral to the centre of the spine.

Function: To disperse wind, promote circulation in the meridian and clear away heat.

2) Shanglian (LI 9)

Location: 3 cun below Quchi (LI 11).

Function: To promote circulation and spread qi.

3) Jugu (LI 16)

Location: In the depression between the acromial extremity of the clavicle and the scapular spine.

Function: To disperse wind and promote circulation in the meridian.

4) Shousanli (LI 10)

Location: On the line joining Yangxi (LI 5) and Quchi (LI 11), 2 cun below Quchi (LI 5).

Function: To regulate qi, stop pain and promote circulation in the meridian and collateral.

5) Quyuan (SI 13)

Location: In the depression of the medial aspect of the suprascapular fossa.

Function: To disperse wind and promote circulation in the meridian.

6) Tiaokou (ST 38)

Location: 2 cun above Xiajuxu (ST 39), midway between Dubi (ST 35) and Jiexi (ST 41).

Function: To promote circulation and eliminate wind.

7) Bingfeng (SI 12)

Location: In the centre of the suprascapular fossa, directly above Tianzong (SI 11). When the arm is lifted, the point is at the site of the depression.

Function: To eliminate wind, activate the

circulation of blood, stop pain and open the orifice.

8) Jianjing (GB 21)

Location: Midway between Dazhui (GV 14) and the acromion.

Function: To promote circulation in the meridian and collateral, expel wind, stop pain, relax the chest and descend the upward perversion of qi.

9) Jianzhen (SI 9)

Location: When the arm hangs down, the point is located 1 cun above the posterior end of the axillary fold.

Function: To relax tendons and promote circulation in the meridian.

10) Jianyu (LI 15)

Location: In the centre of the starting region of m. deltoideus, at the lower border of the clavicular acromion. When the arm is in full abduction, the point is in the depression appearing at the anterior of the shoulder.

Function: To disperse wind and promote circulation in the meridian.

10. Low Back and Spinal Pain.

Yaoshu (GV 2), Hunmen (BL 47), Yinmen (BL 37), Pangguangshu (BL 28), Sanjiaoshu (BL 22), Baliao (BL31-34), Chengshan (BL 57), Chengfu (BL 36), Kunlun(BL 60), Biguan (ST 31), Qihaishu (BL

24), Zhonglushu (BL 29), Huangmen (BL 51), Heyang (BL 55), Zhishi (BL 52), Houxi (SI 3), Dazhui (GV 14), Fuyang (BL 59), Dachangshu (BL 25).

1) Yaoshu (GV 2)

Location: In the hiatus of the sacrum.

Function: To strengthen the lumbus and kidney.

2) Hunmen (BL 47)

Location: 3 cun lateral to the lower border of the spinous process of the 9th thoracic vertebra.

Function: To smooth the liver qi, benefit the gallbladder functions and promote circulation in the meridian and collateral.

3) Yinmen (BL 37)

Location: 6 cun directly below Chengfu (BL 36).

Function: To relax tendons and promote circulation in the meridian and collateral.

4) Pangguangshu (BL 28)

Location:1.5 cun lateral to Governor Vessel, at the lever of the 2nd posterior sacral foramen. In the depression between the medial border of the posterior-superior iliac spine and the sacrum.

Function: To be anti-inflammtion and diuresis.

5) Sanjiaoshu (BL 22)

Location: 1.5 cun lateral to the lower border of the spinous process of the 1st lumber vertebra.

Function: To remove the stagnation of qi from the Triple Energizers.

6) Baliao (BL 31-34)

Location: BL 31, 32, 33 and BL 34 are located in the 1st, 2nd, 3rd and 4th sacral foramens successively.

Function: To regulate the function of the Lower Energizer and strengthen the lumbus and knees.

7) Chengshan (BL 57)

Location: On the posterior of the leg, below the belly of m. gastrocnemius, on the crease of the mark of "人" when the leg is extended.

Function: To activate the circulation of blood, remove the stasis, coolen the mind and relieve spasm.

8) Chengfu (BL 36)

Location: In the middle of the transverse gluteal fold. To locate the point in prone position.

Function: To strengthen the body resistance, eliminate the pathogenic factors, relax tendons and promote circulation in the meridian.

9) Kunlun (BL 60)

Location: In the depression between the external malleolus and tendo calcaneus.

Function: To expel wind, promote circulation in the meridian, relax tendons, strengthen the lumber region and calm down the mind.

10) Biguan (ST 31)

Location: On the anterior aspect of the thigh, directly below the anterior-superior iliac spine, in the depression when the thigh is flexed, opposite to Chengfu (BL 36).

Function: To promote circulation in the meridian and collateral.

11) Qihaishu (BL 24)

Location: 1.5 cun lateral to Governor Vessel, at the level with the lower border of the spinous process of the 3rd lumbar vertebra.

Function: To regulate qi and stop pain.

12) Zhonglushu (BL 29)

Location: 1.5 cun lateral to Governor Vessel, at the level with the 3rd posterior sacral foramen.

Function: To strengthen the lumbus and the kidney functions.

13) Huangmen (BL 51)

Location: 3 cun lateral to the lower border of the spinous process of the 1st lumbar vertebra (the 13th vertebra).

Function: To relax tendons and promote circulation in the meridion.

14) Heyang (BL 55)

Location: Between two heads of m. gastroc-
nemius, on the line joining Weizhong (BL 40) and
Chengshan (BL 57), 2 cun directly below Weizhong
(BL 40).

Function: To regulate the circulation of qi and
blood.

15) Zhishi (BL 52)

Location: 3 cun lateral to the lower border of
the spinous process of the 2nd lumbar vertebra.

Function: To strengthen the lumbus and the
kidney functions.

16) Houxi (SI 3)

Location: When a loose fist is made, the point
is on the ulnar side, proximal to the 5th metacarpophalangeal joint, at the end of the transverse
crease.

Function: To clear away heat, expel wind and
promote circulation of the meridian and collateral.

17) Dazhui (GV 14)

Location: Below the spinous process of the 7th
cervical vertebra.

Function: To dispel wind, clear away heat,
relieve the exterior syndromes and promote the
circulation of yang qi.

18) Fuyang (BL 59)

Location: 3 cun above the external malleolus, between the tendon and bone, anterior to Taiyang meridian and posterior to Shaoyang meridian.

Function: To promote the circulation of qi and remove obstruction.

19) Dachangshu (BL 25)

Location: 1.5 cun lateral to the lower border of the spinous process of the 4th lumbar vertebra, at the level with the upper border of the iliac crest.

Function: To regulate the circulation of qi and stop pain.

11.Pain of the Upper Limbs

Shanglian (LI 9), Tianjing (TE 10), Tianzong (SI 11), Jugu(LI 16), Shaohai (HT 3), Shousanli (LI 10), Shouwuli (LI 13), Waiguan (TE 5), Quchi (LI 11), Houxi (SI 3), Bingfeng (SI 12), Jianliao (TE 14), Jianyu (LI 15), Gaogu (Extra), Binao (LI 14), Shangyang (LI 1).

1) Shanglian (LI 9)

Location: 3 cun below Quchi (LI 11).

Function: To promote circulation in the meridian and collateral and expel the pathogenic factors.

2) Tianjing (TE 10)

Location: In the depression between the two

tendons posterior to the big bone of the lateral side of the elbow, about 1 cun posterior and superior to the olecranon.

Function: To lubricate joints, brighten the eyes and benefit the brain.

3) Tianzong (SI 11)

Location: In the centre of the infrascapular fossa. A triangular shape is almost formed by Naoshu (SI 10), Jianzhen (SI 9) and this point.

Function: To relax tendons and promote circulation in the meridian and collateral.

4) Jugu (LI 16)

Location: In the depression between the acromial extremity of the clavicle and the scapular spine.

Function: To dispel wind and promote circulation in the meridian and collateral.

5) Shaohai (HT 3)

Location: When the elbow is flexed, the point is in medial end of the transverse cubital crease.

Function: To promote circulation in the meridian and collateral.

6) Shousanli (LI 10)

Location: On the line joining Yangxi (LI 5) and Quchi (LI 11), 2 cun below Quchi (LI 11).

Function: To regulate qi circulation, stop pain,

relax tendons and promote circulation in the meridian and collateral.

7) Shouwuli (LI 13)

Location: 3 cun above the elbow, in the center of the triceps muscle of arm, on the medial aspect of the humerus. The point is located when the arm is flexed.

Function: To promote circulation in the meridian and collateral and expel the pathogenic factors.

8) Waiguan (TE 5)

Location: On the dorsum of the forearm, 2 cun posterior to the transverse crease of the wrist, between the radius and ulna.

Function: To dispel heat and eliminate the exterior syndromes, promote circulation in the meridian and collateral.

9) Quchi (LI 11)

Location: When the elbow is flexed, the point is in the depression at the lateral end of the transverse cubital crease.

Function: To expel wind, eliminate the exterior syndromes, clear away heat and regulate nutrients and blood.

10) Houxi (SI 3)

Location: When a loose fist is made, the point

is on the ulnar side, at the end of the transverse crease posterior to the 5th metacarpophalangeal joint.

Function: To clear away heat, eliminate wind and promote circulation in the meridian and collateral.

11) Bingfeng (SI 12)

Location: In the centre of the suprascapular fossa, directly above Tianzong (SI 11). When the arm is lifted, the point is at the site of the depression.

Function: To expel wind, activate the circulation of blood, stop pain and open the orifice.

12) Jianliao (TE 14)

Location: About 1 cun posterior to Jianyu (LI 15), in the depression posterior and inferior to the acromion.

Function: To promote circulation in the meridian and collateral, disperse wind and open the orifice.

13) Jianyu (LI 15)

Location: In the middle of the beginning region of m. deltoideus, at the inferior border of the acromioclavicle, in the depression appearing anterior to the shoulder when the arm is fully abduction.

Function: To promote circulation in the meridian and disperse wind.

14) Gaogu (Extra)

Location: Anterior to Cun region and posterior to the palm. The point is located bilaterally superior to the condyle of the radius.

Function: To ease pain and stop spasm.

15) Binao (LI 14)

Location: On the line joining Quchi (LI 11) and Jianyu (LI 15), 7 cun above the elbow, on the lateral aspect of the humerus and the lower end of m. detoideus.

Function: To promote circulation in the meridian and collateral, clear away heat and brighten the eyes.

16) Shangyang (LI 1)

Location: On the radial side of the index finger, about 0.1 cun posterior to the corner of the nail.

Function: To ease pain and clear away heat.

12. Hypochondriac Pain

Yanglingquan (GB 34), Dabao (SP 21), Zhigou (TE 6), Yunmen (LU 2), Riyue (GB 24), Xingjian (LR 2) Yangfu (GB 38), Jiquan (HT 1), Qimen (LR 14) Qingling (HT 2).

1) Yanglingquan (GB 34)

Location: Inferior to the lateral side of the knee joint, in the depression anterior and inferior to the head of the fibula.

Function: To promote circulation in the meridian and collateral, smooth the liver qi and benefit the gallbladder functions and eliminate damp and heat.

2) Dabao (SP 21)

Location: Directly below the mid-axillary line, in the 6th intercostal space.

Function: To promote circulation in the meridian and collateral.

3) Zhigou (TE 6)

Location: On the flexion aspect of the forearm, 3 cun posterior to the wrist, between the ulna and radius.

Function: To promote circulation in the meridian and collateral, descend the upward perversion of qi and smooth the liver qi.

4) Yunmen (LU 2)

Location: Inferior to the lateral end of the clavicle, between the upper border of m. pectoralis major and the clavicle.

Function: To relax the chest and release asthma.

5) Riyue (GB 24)

Location: One rib below Qimen (LR 14) in the 7th intercostal space.

Function: To regulate qi circulation and stop pain.

6) Xingjian (LR 2)

Location: On the dorsum of the foot between the 1st and 2nd toes, in the depression about 0.5 cun posterior to the margin of the web.

Function: To promote circulation in the meridian and collateral and smooth the liver qi.

7) Yangfu (GB 38)

Location: 4 cun above the tip of the external malleolus, slightly anterior to the anterior border of the fibula.

Function: To promote circulation in the meridian and collateral and eliminate wind and damp

8) Jiquan (HT 1)

Location: In the centre of the axilla, on the medial side of the axillary artery.

Function: To ease pain and activate the circulation of blood.

9) Qimen (LR 14)

Location: On the midline of the nipple, in the 2 nd intercostal space below the nipple or in the 6th intercostal space.

Function: To relax the chest, promote the

circulation of qi, relieve inflammation and stop pain.

10) Qingling (HT 2)

Location: 3 cun above Shaohai (HT 3).

Function: To promote circulation in the meridian and collateral.

13. Lower Limb Pain

Huantiao (GB 30), Yanglingquan (GB 34), Weizhong (BL 40), Kunlun (BL 60), Zusanli (ST 36), Xiaochangshu (BL 27), Pushen (BL 61), Fengshi (GB 31), Guangming (GB 37), Heyang (BL 55), Chongyang (ST 42), Tiaokou(ST 38), Mingmen (GV 4), Juliao (GB 29), Fuliu(KI 7), Yaoyangguan (GV 3), Jiexi (ST 41), Xiajuxu(St 39), Baliao (BL31-BL34), Xiyangguan (GB 33), Chengfu (BL 36), Zhibian (BL 54), Yongquan (KI 1), Fuyang (BL 59)

1) Huantiao (GB 30)

Location: In the depression posterior and superior to the great trochanter.

Function: To promote circulation in the meridian and collateral, eliminate wind and cold and strengthen the lumbar and legs.

2) Yanglingquan (GB 34)

Location: In the depression anterior and inferior to the head of the fibula, on the lateral inferior aspect of the knee joint.

Function: To promote circulation in the meridian and collateral, eliminate damp and heat, smooth the liver qi and benefit the gallbadder functions.

3) Weizhong (BL 40)

Location: Midpoint of the transverse crease of the popliteal fossa.

Function:To regulate qi, promote the circulation in the meridian and collateral, reduce summer heat. It is the point for sudden onset of Wei and Bi syndromes of the lower limbs.

4) Kunlun(BL 60)

Location: In the depression between the tip of the external malleclus and tendo calcaneus.

Function: To expel wind, promote circulation in the meridian, relax tendons and strengthen the lumbus.

5) Zusanli (ST 36)

Location: 3 cun below the lower border of the patella and one finger-breadth lateral to the anterior crest of the tibia.

Function: To calm down the mind, stop pain, tonify qi and blood, regulate the circulation of qi and blood and readjust the functions of the spleen and stomach.

6) Xiaochangshu (BL 27)

Location: 1.5 cun lateral to Governor Vessel, at the level with the 1st posterior sacral foramen. In the depression between the medial border of the posterior-superior iliac spine and sacrum.

Function: To regulate the digestive tract.

7) Pushen (BL 61)

Location: Posterior and inferior to the external malleolus, directly below Kunlun (BL 60), in the depression of calcaneum.

Function: To promote the circulation of blood and expel wind.

8) Fengshi (GB 31)

Location:On the midline of the lateral aspect of the thigh, about 7 cun above the patella. When the patient is standing erect with the hands close to the sides, the point is where the tip of the middle finger touches.

Function: To promote circulation of the meridian and collateral, and eliminate wind and damp.

9) Guangming (GB 37)

Location: 5 cun directly above the tip of the external malleolus, on the anterior border of the fibula, between m. flexor digitorum longus pedis and m. peroneus brevis.

Function: To remove stagnation, eliminate heat and relieve pain in the lower extremities.

10) Heyang (BL 55)

Location:2 cun directly below Weizhong (BL 40), between medial and lateral heads of m. gastrocnemius, on the line joining Weizhong (BL 40) and Chengshan (BL 57).

Function: To promote the circulation of qi and blood.

11) Chongyang (ST 42)

Location: 1.5 cun below Jiexi (ST 41), in the depression between the 2nd and 3rd metatarsal bones and the cuneiform bone.

Function: To promote the circulation of blood in the meridian and treat paralysis of the lower extremities.

12) Tiaokou (ST 38)

Location: The midpoint on the line joining Dubi (ST 35) and Jiexi (ST 41), 2 cun below Xiajuxu (ST 37).

Function: To promote circulation and expel wind.

13) Mingmen (GV 4)

Location: Below the 22nd vertebra, between the spinous processes of the 2nd and 3rd lumbar vertebras.

Function: To strengthen yang, benefit qi activity, lubricate lumbar region, tonify the kidney functions and calm down the mind.

14) Juliao (GB 29)

Location: In the depression of the midpoint between the anteriosuperior iliac spine and the great trochanter.

Function: To promote circulation in the lumbar region and legs.

15) Fuliu (KI 7)

Location: In the depression, 2 cun above the medial malleolus.

Function: To develop yang, eliminate the exterior syndromes and relieve leg swelling.

16) Yaoyangguan (GV 3)

Location: Below the spinous process of the 4th lumbar vertebra, at the level with the crista iliaca.

Function: To strengthen the kidney yang, regulate the circulation of qi and blood.

17) Jiexi (ST 41)

Location: In the depression of the midpoint of the transverse crease between the dorsum of the foot and the leg.

Function: To promote circulation in the meridian and collateral and conduct the stagnated heat in the Upper Energizer transforing downward.

18) Xiajuxu (ST 39)

Location:3 cun below Shangjuxu (ST 37), one

finger-breadth from the anterior crest of the tibia.

Function: To tranquilize the mind and stop pain.

19) Baliao (BL 31 to BL 34)

Location: BL 31, 32, 33 and 34 are located in the 1st, 2nd, 3rd and 4th sacral foramens successively.

Function: To regulate the functions in the Lower Energizer, and strengthen the lumbar•and knees.

20) Xiyangguan (GB 33)

Location: 3 cun above Yanglingquan (GB 34), in the depression of the lateral-superior border of the femur.

Function: To promote circulation in the meridian and collateral, and disperse wind and cold.

21) Chengfu (BL⁻36)

Location:In the middle of the transverse gluteal fold. To locate the point in prone position.

Function: To strengthen the antipathogenic qi, eliminate the pathogenic factors, relax tendons and promote circulation in the meridian and collateral.

22) Zhibian (BL 54)

Location:3 cun lateral to the lower border of the spinous process of the 4 th sacral vertebra.

Function: To promote circulation in the meridian and collateral.

23) Yongquan (KI 1)

Location: On the sole, in the depression when the foot is in plantar flexion.

Function:To promote circulation in the meridian and collateral, nourish yin to reduce fire and nourish the liver functions to eliminate wind.

24) Fuyang (BL 59)

Location: 3 cun above the external malleolus, between the tendon and bone, in front of Taiyang meridian and behind Shaoyang meridian.

Function:To promote the circulation of qi and remove obstruction.

14. Pain of the Wrist Joint

Daling (PC 7), Yangchi (TE 4), Lieque (LU 7), Yangxi (LI 5), Ximen (PC 4), Gaogu (Extra).

1) Daling (PC 7)

Location:Posterior to the palm, in the middle of the transverse crease of the wrist.

Function: To stop pain.

2) Yangchi (TE 4)

Location:On the transverse crease of the dorsum of the wrist, on the ulna side of the tendon of m. extensor digitorum communis.

Function: To lubricate the joint.

3) Lieque (LU 7)

Location: Superior to the styloid proeess of the radius, 1.5 cun above the transverse crease of the wirst.

Function: To promote circulation in the meridian and collateral.

4) Yangxi (LI 5)

Location: On the dorsum of the wirst, in the depression between the tendons of m. extensor pollicis longus and brevis.

Function: To activate the circulation of qi and blood, disperse wind and clear away heat.

5) Ximen (PC 4)

Location: In the centre of the palmar side of the forearm, 5 cun posterior to the transverse crease of the wrist, in the depression between the two tendons.

Function: To relax tendons and promote circulation in the meridian.

6) Gaogu (Extra)

Location:Posterior to the palm and anterior to Cun region, one point on each side of the supracondyle of the radia.

Function:To ease pain and stop spasm.

15.Knee Joint Pain

Xiguan (LR 7), Weizhong (BL 40), Xuanzhong (GB 39), Xiyangguan (GB 33), Tiaokou (ST 38),

Yingu (KI 10), Biguan (ST 31), Pushen (BL 61), Fengshi (GB 31), Zusanli (ST 36), Ququan (LR 8), Futu (ST 32), Yangjiao (GB 35), Yanglingquan (GB 34), Xiyan (Ex-LE4) on both sides of the knee joint.

1) Xiguan (LR 7)

Location: 7 cun above the tip of the medial malleolus, 1 cun posterior to Yinlingquan (SP 9)

Function: To disperse wind to eliminate cold.

2) Weizhong (BL 40)

Location: Midpoint of the transverse crease of the popliteal fossa.

Function: To promote circulation in the meridian and collateral and regulate qi functions.

3) Xuanzhong (GB 39)

Location: 3 cun above the tip of the external malleolus slightly anterior to the fibula, in the broken-like place of the bone by the touching of the thomb.

Function: To disperse wind, eliminate damp and promote circulation in the meridian and collateral.

4) Xiyangguan (GB 33)

Location: 3 cun above Yanglingquan (GB 34), in the depression of the lateral and superior border of the femur.

Function:To promote circulation of the meridian and collateral and eliminate wind and cold.

5) Tiaokou (ST 38)

Location: 2 cun above Xiajuxu (ST 39), midway between Dubi (ST 35) and Jiexi (ST 41).

Function: To keep free circulation and eliminate wind.

6) Yingu (KI 10)

Location: When the knee is flexed, the point is on the medial side of the popliteal fossa, between the tendons of m. semitendinosus and sememembranosus, at the level with Weizhong (BL 40).

Function: To strengthen the lumbus and knee joints.

7) Biguan (ST 31)

Location: In front of the thigh, directly below the superior and inferior iliac spine, in the depression when the thigh is flexed, and corresponding to Chengfu (BL 36).

Function: To promote circulation in the meridian and collaleral.

8) Pushen (BL 61)

Location:Posterior and inferior to the external malleolus, directly below Kunlun (BL 60), in the depression of the calcaneum.

Function: To promote the circulation of blood and eliminate wind.

9) Fengshi (GB 31)

Location: On the midline of the lateral aspect of the thigh, 7 cun above the transverse popliteal crease. When the patient is standing erect with the hands close to the sides, the point is where the tip of the middle finger touches.

Function: To promote circulation in the meridian and collateral and eliminate wind and damp.

10) Zusanli (ST 36)

Location: 3 cun below the lower border of the patella, one finger-breadth from the anterior crest of the tibia.

Function: To stop pain, calm down the mind, regulate the circulation of qi and blood and tonify qi and nourish blood.

11) Ququan (LR 8)

Location: When knee is flexed, the point is in the depression above the medial end of the transverse popliteal crease, posterior to the medial epicondyle of the femur.

Function: To promote circulation in the meridian and collateral.

12) Futu (ST 32)

Location: 6 cun above the upper border of the patella when the knee is flexed. On the line connecting the anterior and superior iliac spine and superior lateral border of the patella. The point is on the highest region of the muscle when the leg is forcefully extended.

Function:To relax tendons and promote circulation of the meridian.

13) Yangjiao (GB 35)

Location:6 cun above the tip of the external malleolus, on the line joining the tip of the external malleolus and Yinlingquan (SP 9).

Function: To remove stagnation, relieve spasm and treat knee pain.

14) Yanglingquan (GB 34)

Location: Below the lateral side of the knee joint, in the depression anterior and inferior to the head of the fibula.

Function: To promote circulation in the meridian and collateral.

15) Xiyan (Ex-LE4)

Location: A pair of points in the two depressions, medial and lateral to the patellar ligaments.

Function: To relax tendons, promote the circulation of blood in the meridian and collateral, disperse wind and cold, ease pain and stop spasm.

16.Pain of the Ankle

Jinmen (BL 63), Kunlun (BL 60), Jiexi (ST 41), Tiaokou (ST 38), Fuyang (BL 59).

1) Jinmen (BL 63)

Location: Below the external malleolus, 0.5 cun anterior to Shenmai (BL 62).

Function: To eliminate wind, promote circulation in the meridian and collateral.

2) Kunlun (BL 60)

Location: In the depression between the external malleolus and tendo caloaneus.

Function: To expel wind, promote circulation in the meridian and collateral, relax tendons and strengthen the lumbus.

3) Jiexi (ST 41)

Locaiton: On the dorsum of the foot, in the depression of the midpoint of the transverse crease of the ankle joint.

Function: To promote circulation in the meridian and collateral and conduct the stagnated heat in the Upper Enerziger going downward.

4) Tiaokou (ST 38)

Location: 2 cun above Xiajuxu (ST 39), midway between Dubi (ST 35) and Jiexi (ST 41).

Function: To keep free circulation and expel wind.

5) Fuyang (BL 59)

Location: 3 cun above the external malleolus, between the tendon and bone, in front of Taiyang meridian and behind Shaoyang meridian.

Function: To promote the circulation of qi and remove obstruction.

17. Rheumatoid Arthritis

Hegu (LI 4), Zusanli (ST 36), Diwuhui (GB 42), Fengshi (GB 31), Quchi (LI 11), Weizhong (BL 40), swelling and pain regions.

1) Hegu (LI 4)

Location: On the dorsum of the hand, between the 1st and 2nd metacarpal bones approximately in the middle of the 2nd metacarpal bones on the radial side.

Function: To disperse wind, eliminate the exterior syndromes, promote the circulation of qi and blood in the meridian and collateral and stop pain.

2) Zusanli (ST 36)

Location: 3 cun below the lower border of the patella, one finger-breadth from the anterior crest of the tibia.

Function: To stop pain, calm down the mind, regulate the circulation of qi and blood, tonify qi and nourish blood, and regulate the functions of the spleen and stomach.

3) Diwuhui (GB 42)

Location: Between the 4th and 5th metatarsal

bones, on the medial side of the tendon of m. extensor digiti minimi of foot.

Funtion: To promote circulation in the meridian and collateral, disperse wind and open the orifice.

4) Fengshi (GB 31)

Location: On the midline of the lateral aspect of the thigh, 7 cun above the transverse popliteal crease. When the patient is standing erect with the hands close to the sides, the point is where the tip of the middle finger touches.

Funtion: To promote circulation in the meridian and collateral and eliminate wind and damp.

5) Quchi (LI 11)

Location: When the elbow is flexed, the point is in the depression at the lateral end of the transverse cubital crease.

Funtion: To expel wind, eliminate the exterior syndromes, clear away heat and harmonize nutrient and blood systems.

6) Weizhong (BL 40)

Location: Midpoint of the transverse crease of the popliteal fossa.

Function: To regulate qi, promote the circulation of blood in the meridian.

18.Hypertension

Neiguan (PC 6), Yongquan (KI 1), Renying (ST 9), Sanyinjiao (SP 6), Taichong (LR 3), Baihui (GV 20), Hegu (LI 4), Zusanli (ST 36), Yinbai (SP 1).

1) Neiguan (PC 6)

Location: 2 cun above the transverse crease of the wrist, between the tendons of m. palmaris longus and m. flexor radialis.

Function: To calm down the mind, relax the chest, descend the upward perversion of qi, harmonize the Middle Energizer and stop pain.

2) Yongquan (KI 1)

Location: On the sole, in the depression when the foot is in plantar flexion.

Function: To promote circulation in the meridian and collateral, nourish yin to reduce fire, nourish the liver to pacify wind, open the orifice and calm down the mind.

3) Renying (ST 9)

Location: 1.5 cun lateral to the tip of Adam's apple, on the anterior border of m. sternocleidomastoideus. To avoid to the artery during puncturing.

Function: To dispel wind and promote circulation in the collateral.

4) Sanyinjiao (SP 6)

Location: 3 cun directly above the tip of the

medial malleolus, on the posterior border of the medial aspect of the tibia.

Function: To strengthen the spleen functions so as to resolve damp, smooth the liver qi, benefit the kidney functions, nourish yin to moisten dryness.

5) Taichong (LR 3)

Location: On the dorsum of the foot, in the depression distal to the junction of the 1st and 2nd metatarsal bones.

Function: To regulate the liver qi, activate the circulation of blood and remove stagnation.

6) Baihui (GV 20)

Location: In the centre of the vertex, 5 cun posterior to the anterior hairline and 7 cun anterior to the posterior hairline.

Function: To clear away heat and open the orifice, elevate yang to treat the prolapse and calm down the mind.

7) Hegu (LI 4)

Location: On the dorsum of the hand, between the 1st and 2nd metacarpal bones, approximately in the middle of the 2nd metacarpal bone on the radial side.

Function: To disperse wind, eliminate the exterior syndromes, promote the circulation of qi

and blood in the meridian and collateral and stop
pain.

8) Zusanli (ST 36)

Location: 3 cun below the lower border of the
patella, one finger-breadth from the anterior crest
of the tibia.

Function: To tonify and nourish qi and blood,
calm down the mind, stop pain and regulate the
circulation of qi and blood.

9) Yinbai (SP 1)

Location: On the medial side of the great toe,
0.1 cun posterior to the corner of the nail.

Function: To benefit the spleen functions to
regulate the blood circulation.

19. Cardiac Disorders

Xinshu (BL 15), Neiguan (PC 6), Shaochong
(HT 9), Shaoze (SI 1), Shaohai (HT 3),Juque (CV
14), Zhongchong (PC 9), Yinxi (HT 6), Jiuwei (CV
15), Jianshi (PC 5), Shenmen (HT 7), Jueyinshu (BL
14), Daling (PC 7), Taiyi (ST 23), Quze (PC 3),
Guanchong (TE 1), Laogong (PC 8), Huangmen (BL
51), Tongli (HT 5), Dushu(BL 16).

1) Xinshu (BL 15)

Location: 1.5 cun lateral to the lower border of
the spinous process of the 5th thoracic vertebra.

Function: To tranquilize the mind.

2) Neiguan (PC 6)

Location: 2 cun above the transverse crease of the wrist, on the medial aspect of the forearm, in the depression between the two tendons.

Function: To calm down the mind, relax the chest and descend the upward perversion of qi, harmonize the Middle Energizer and stop pain.

3) Shaochong (HT 9)

Location: On the radial side of the little finger, about 0.1 cun posterior to the corner of the nail.

Function: To calm down the mind, promote the circulation of qi in the meridian.

4) Shaoze (SI 1)

Location: On the ulnar side of the little finger, about 0.1 cun posterior to the corner of the nail.

Function: To clear away heat and moisten dryness.

5) Shaohai (HT 3)

Location: When the elbow is flexed into a right angle, the point is in the depression at the medial end of the transverse cubital crease.

Function: To promote circulation in the meridian and collateral.

6) Juque (CV 14)

Location: On the midline of the abdomen, 6 cun above the umbilicus.

Function: To descend the upward perversion of Zang qi.

7) Zhongchong (PC 9)

Location: In the centre of the tip of the middle finger.

Function: To rescue yang from the collapse, open the orifice, and promote circulation in the meridian. It is one of the important points for the emergency.

8) Yinxi (HT 6)

Location: On the radiel side of the tendon of m. flexor carpi ulnaris, 0.5 cun above the transverse crease of the wrist.

Function: To calm down the mind and promote circulation in the meridian and collateral.

9) Jiuwei (CV 15)

Location: Below the xiphoid process, 7 cun above the umbilicus; to locate the point in supine position with the arms uplifted.

Function: To calm down the mind, regulate qi circulation and stop pain.

10) Jianshi (PC 5)

Location: 3 cun above the transverse crease of the wirst, between the tendons of m. palmaris longus and m. flexor carpi radialis.

Function: To calm down the mind and promote

circulation of the meridian and collateral.

11) Shenmen (HT 7)

Location: In the depression of the ulnar end of the transverse crease of the wrist. To avoid to the artery during puncturing.

Function: To calm down the mind and promote circulation of the meridian and collateral.

12) Jueyinshu (BL 14)

Location: 1.5 cun lateral to the lower border of the spinous process of the 4th thoracic vertebra.

Function: To rescue yang from the collapse.

13) Daling (PC 7)

Location: In the middle of the transverse crease of the wrist, between the two tendons.

Function: To calm down the mind and treat insomnia.

14) Taiyi (ST 23)

Location: 2 cun above the umbilicus, 2 cun lateral to Xiawan (CV 10).

Function: To calm down the mind and ease pain.

15) Quze (PC 3)

Location: On the transverse cubital crease, at the ulnar side of the tendon of m. biceps brachi.

Function: To ease fright and release pain.

16) Guanchong (TE 1)

Location: On the lateral side of the ring finger, about 0.1 cun posterior to the corner of the nail.

Function: To clear away fire from the Triple Energizers, eliminate heat and ease pain.

17) Laogong (PC 8)

Location: On the transverse crease of the palm, between the 2nd and 3rd metacarpal bones, When the fist is clenched, the point is just below the tip of the middle finger.

Function: To nourish yin and calm down the mind.

18) Huangmen (BL 51)

Locaiton: 3 cun lateral to the lower border of the spinous process of 1st lumber vertebra (the 13th vertebra).

Function: To relax tendons and promote circulation in the meridian and collateral.

19) Tongli (HT 5)

Location: 1 cun above the transverse crease of the wrist, on the radial side of the tendon of m. flexor carpi ulnaris.

Function: To calm down the mind and promote circulation in the meridian and collateral.

20) Dushu (BL 16)

Location: 1.5 cun lateral to the lower border of the spinous process of the 6th thoracic vertebra.

Function: To regulate qi circulation and stop pain.

20. Tracheitis

Tiantu (CV 22), Yuji (LU 10), Zhongfu (LU 1), Fenglong (ST 40), Gaohuangshu (BL 43), Xuanji (CV 21), Shaoshang (LU 11), Renying (ST 9), Neiguan (PC 6), Fengmen (BL 12), Kufang (ST 14), Feishu (BL 13), Zigong (CV 19), Pohu (BL 42).

1)Tiantu (CV 22)

Location: In the centre of the suprasternal fossa.

Function: To descend the upward perversion of qi and stop cough.

2)Yuji (LU 10)

Location: On the radial aspect of the midpoint of the 1st metacarpal bone, on the junction of the red and white skin.

Function: To stop cough and release asthma.

3) Zhongfu (LU 1)

Location: Laterosuperior to the sternum at the lateral side of the 1st intercostal space, 6 cun lateral to the anterior midline and about 1 cun directly below Yunmen (LU 2).

Function: To remove stagnation, stop cough and relieve asthma.

4) Fenglong (ST 40)

Location: 8 cun above the external malleolus, midway between the lower border of the patellar and the external malleolus.

Function: To clear the mind, smooth the circulation of qi and conduct yang flowing upward.

5) Gaohuangshu (BL 43)

Location: 3 cun lateral to the lower border of the spinous process of the 4th thoracic vertebra.

Function: To calm down the mind and rescue yang from the collapse.

6) Xuanji (CV 21)

Location: On the anterior midline, at the level with the 1st intercostal space.

Function: To reduce the upward perversion of qi and stop cough.

7) Shaoshang (LU 11)

Location: On the radial side of the thumb, about 0.1 cun posterior to the corner of the nail.

Function: To moisten the lung and stop cough.

8) Renying (ST 9)

Location: Level with the tip of Adam's apple, on the anterior border of m. sternocleidomastoideus. To avoid to the artery during puncturing.

Function: To expel wind and promote circulation in the meridian and collateral.

9) Neiguan (PC 6)

Locaiton: 2 cun above the transverse crease of the wrist, between the tendons of m. palmaris longus and m. flexor radialis.

Function: To relax the chest, reduce the upward perversion of qi, calm down the mind, harmonize the Middle Energizer and stop pain.

10) Fengmen (BL 12)

Location: 1.5 cun lateral to the lower border of the spinous process of the 2nd thoracic vertebra.

Function: To disperse wind and regulate the lung qi.

11) Kufang (ST 14)

Location: In the 1st intercostal space, on the midline of the nipple.

Function: To harmonize the Middle Energizer and regulate qi circulation.

12) Feishu (BL 13)

Location: 1.5 cun lateral to the lower border of the spinous process of the 3rd thoracic vertebra.

Function: To stop pain, relieve asthma and regulate the lung qi.

13) Zigong (CV 19)

Location: On the anterior midline, at the level with the 2nd intercostal space.

Function: To ease cough and relieve asthma.

14)Pohu (BL 42)

Location: 3 cun lateral to the lower border of the spinous process of the 3rd thoracic vertebra.

Function: To disperse qi and remove stagnation.

21. Common Cold

Dazhui (GV 14), Fengchi (GB 20), Taodao (GV 13), Dazhu (BL 11), Shangxing (GV 23), Tianzhu (BL 10), Tongtian (BL 7), Kongzui (LU 6), Fengmen (BL 12), Waiguan (TE 6), Baihui (GV 20), Houxi (SI 3), Hegu (LI 4), Yangchi (TE 4), Jiaosun (TE 20), Qingling (HT 2), Jianjing (GB 21), Chengling (GB 18), Wangu (SI 4).

1) Dazhui (GV 14)

Location: Below the spinous process of the 7th cervical vertebra.

Function: To disperse wind, clear away heat, eliminate the exterior syndromes,promote yang circulation, clear and calm down the mind.

2)Fengchi (GB 20)

Location: On the back of the nape, in the depression between m. sternocleidomastoideus and the upper portion of m. trapezius, below the occiput.

Function: To disperse wind, clear away heat, promote circulation in the meridian and collateral. brighten the eyes and open the orifice.

3) Taodao (GV 13)

Location: Below the spinous process of the 1st thoracic vertebra.

Function: To clear away heat and expel wind.

4) Dazhu (BL 11)

Location: 1.5 cun lateral to the lower border of the spinous process of the 1st thoracic vertebra.

Function: To disperse wind, promote circulation in the meridian and collateral and clear away heat.

5) Shangxing (GV 23)

Locaiton: One cun within the anterior hairline and 4 cun anterior to Baihui (GV 20).

Function: To clear the mind and brighten eyes.

6) Tianzhu (BL 10)

Location: 1.3 cun lateral to Yamen (GV 15), on the lateral aspect of m. trapezius.

Function: To treat dizziness and open the orifice.

7) Tongtian (BL 7)

Locaiton: 1.5 cun posterior to Chengguang (BL 6).

Function: To connect to qi of the heaven, by the point, qi in Foot-Taiyang meridian is conducted up to the vertex at Baihui (GV 20).

.8) Kongzui (LU 6)

Locaiton: On the line joining Chize (LU 5) and Taiyuan (LU 9), 5 cun below Chize (LU 5) and 7 cun above Taiyuan (LU 9).

Function: To clear away heat, ease pain, and relieve asthma and cough.

9) Fengmen (BL 12)

Location: 1.5 cun lateral to the lower border of the spinous process of the 2nd thoracic vertebra.

Function: To disperse wind and regulate the lung qi.

10) Waiguan (TE 5)

Location: On the dorsum of the forearm, 2 cun posterior to the transverse crease of the wrist, between the radius and ulna.

Function: To eliminate the exterior syndromes, clear away heat and promote circulation in the meridian and collateral.

11) Baihui (GV 20)

Location: In the centre of the vertex, 5 cun posterior to the anterior hairline and 7 cun anterior to the posterior hairline.

Function: To clear away heat, open the orifice, elevate yang for the prolapse, pacify the liver yang and calm down the mind.

12) Houxi (SI 3)

Location: When a loose fist is made, the point

is on the ulnar side, proximal to the 5th metacarpophalangeal joint, at the end of the transverse crease.

Function: To clear away heat, eliminate wind and promote circulation in the meridian and collateral.

13) Hegu (LI 4)

Location: On the dorsum of the hand, between the 1st and 2nd metacarpal bones, approximately in the middle of the 2nd metacarpal bone on the radial side.

Function: To disperse wind, eliminate the exterior syndromes, open the orifice, promote the circulation of qi and blood in the meridian and collateral and stop pain.

14) Yangchi (TE 4)

Location: On the transverse crease of the dorsum of the wrist, on the ulnar side of the tendon of m. extensor digitorum communis.

Function: To lubricate joints, brighten the eyes and benefit the intelligence.

15) Jiaosun (TE 20)

Location: Directly above the ear apex, within the hairline.

Function: To disperse wind and fire.

16. Qingling (HT 2)

Location: On the medial aspect of the elbow, 3 cun above Shaohai (HT 3).

Function: To promote circulation of the meridian and collateral.

17) Jianjing (GB 21)

Location: Midway between Dazhui (GV 14) and and acromion.

Function: To promote circulation in the meridian and collateral, eliminate wind, stop pain, reduce the upward perversion of qi and relax the chest.

18) Chengling (GB 18)

Location: 1.5 cun posterior to Zhengying (GB 17), on the line connecting Toulinqi (GB 15) and Fengchi (GB 20).

Function: To disperse wind, clear away heat and promote circulation in the meridian and collateral.

19) Wangu (SI 4)

Location: In the depression between the base of the 5th metacarpal bone and the triquetral bone. The point is located when the fist is made.

Function: To disperse wind and promote circulation in the meridian and collateral.

22.Asthmatic Breathing

Tiantu (CV 22), Tanzhong (CV 17), Huagai (CV

20), Xuanji (CV 21), Zhiyang (GV 9), Yuzhong (KI 26), Quepen (ST 12), Dabao (SP 21), Tianfu (LU 3), Zhongfu (LU 1), Qihu (ST 13), Qishe (ST 11), Kongzui (LU 6), Bulang (KI 22), Shenzhu (GV 12), Lingtai (GV 10), Lingxu (KI 24), Pohu (BL 42), Xiabai (LU 4), Feishu (BL 13), Yuji (LU 10), Wuyi (ST 15), Zigong (CV 19), Gaohuangshu (BL 43), Fengmen (BL 12), Renying (ST 9).

1)Tiantu (CV 22)

Location: In the centre of the suprasternal fossa.

Function: To reduce the upward perversion of qi and stop pain.

2) Tanzhong (CV 17)

Location: On the anterior midline, in the depression of the midway between the nipples.

Function: To regulate qi activity, reduce the upward perversion of qi, relax the chest and benefit the diaphragm.

3) Huagai (CV 20)

Location: On the anterior midline, at the level with the lst intercostal space.

Function: To relax the chest, regulate qi activity,reduce the upward perversion of qi and benefit the diaphragm.

4) Xuanji (CV 21)

Location: On the anterior midline, at the level with the lst intercostal space, slightly superior to Huagai (CV 20).

Function: To reduce the upward perversion of qi and stop cough.

5) Zhiyang (GV 9)

Location: Below the spinous process of the thoracic vertebra, approximately at the level with the inferior angle of the scapula.

Function:To treat cough and asthma.

6) Yuzhong (KI 26)

Location: In the lst intercostal space,2 cun lateral to the anterior midline.

Function: To clear away heat,eliminate damp and resolve phlegm.

7) Quepen (ST 12)

Location: Directly below the midpoint of the supraclaviculer fossa, 4 cun lateral to Tiantu(CV 22).

Function:To promote the circulation of qi.

8) Dabao (SP 21)

Location:Directly below the mid-axillary line, in the 6th intercostal space.

Function: To promote circulation in the meridian and collateral.

9) Tianfu (LU 3)

Location: 3 cun below the end of axillary fold, on the radial side of m. biceps brachii, on the medial aspect of the upper arm.

Function: To promote circulation in the meridien and callateral.

10) Zhongfu(LU 1)

Location: Laterosuperior to the sternum, at the lateral side of the lst intercostal space, 6 cun lateral to the anterior midline, 1 cun directly below Yunmen(LU 2).

Function: To remove stagnation, relieve cough and asthma.

11) Qihu (ST 13)

Location: Inferior to the middle of the clavicle, on the superior border of the lst rib, directly opposing to the midline of the nipple.

Function: To relax the chest, regulate the circulation of qi and relieve cough and asthma.

12) Qishe(ST 11)

Location:Directly below Renying (ST 9),at the superior border of the medial end of the clavicular head of m. sternodeidomastoideus.

Function: To descend the upward perversion of qi, regulate qi circulation, activate the circulation of blood and remove stagnation.

13) Kongzui (LU 6)

Location: On the palmar aspect of the forearm, on the line joining Taiyuan(LU9) and Chize(LU5), 5 cun below Chize (LU5), or 7 cun above Taiyuan(LU 9).

Function: To relieve cough and asthma, eliminate heat and ease pain.

14) Bulang (KI 22)

Location:In the 5th intercostal space, 2 cun lateral to Conception Vessel.

Function: To relax the chest, regulate the circulation of qi and reduce the upward perversion of the liver qi.

15) Shenzhu (GV 12)

Location: Below the spinous process of the 3rd thoracic vertebra.

Function: To strengthen the body resistance.

16) Lingtai (GV 10)

Location:Below the spinous process of the 6th thoracic vertebra.

Function:To disperse wind, clear away heat and calm down the mind.

17) Lingxu (KI 24)

Location:In the 3rd intercostal space, 2 cun lateral to the anterior midline.

Function:To benefit the kidney functions, reduce the upward perversion of qi and mainly treat cough and asthma.

18) Pohu(BL 42)

Location: 3 cun lateral to the lower border of the spinous process of the 3rd thoracic vertebra.

Function:To disperse qi and remove stagnation.

19) Xiabai (LU 4)

Location:5 cun above the transverse cubital crease, on the radial side of m. biceps brachii.

Function:To promote the circulation of qi.

20) Feishu (BL 13)

Location:1.5 cun lateral to the lower border of the spinous process of the 3rd thoracic vertebra.

Function:To regulate the lung qi and relieve cough and asthma.

21) Yuji (LU 10)

Location:On the radial aspect of the midpoint of the lst metacarpal bone, on the junction of the red and white skin.

Function:To ease cough and relieve asthma.

22) Wuji(ST 15)

Location:In the 2nd intercostal space, 4 cun lateral to the anterior midline.

Function:To clear away heat and relieve pain.

23) Zigong(CV 19)

Location:On the anterior midline, at the level

with the 2nd intercostal space.

Function:To ease cough and relieve asthma.

24) Gaohuangshu(BL 43)

Location: 3 cun lateral to the lower border of the spinous process of the 4th thoracic vertebra.

Function:To calm down the mind, benefit the intelligence, and rescue yang from the collapse.

25) Fengmen(BL 12)

Location:1.5 cun lateral to the lower border of the spinous process of the 2nd thoracic vertebra.

Function:To disperse wind and regulate the lung qi .

26) Renying(ST 9)

Location:1.5 cun lateral to the tip of Adam's apple on the anterior border of m. sternocleidomastoideus. To avoid to the artery during puncturing.

Function:To expel wind and promote circulation in the meridian and collateral.

23.Gastric Disorder, Dyspepsia,

Shangwan (CV 13), Zhongwan (CV 12), Xiawan (CV 10), Burong (ST 19), Taiyi (ST 23), Zhangmen (LR 13), Taibai (SP 3), Zhongting (CV 16), Yishe (BL 49), Juque (CT 14), Neiguan (PC 6), Gongsun (SP 4), Quze (PC 3), Hegu (LI 4), Guanmen (ST 22), Zusanli (ST 36), Jianshi (PC 5), Fuai (SP 16), Lingxu(KI 24), Jianli (CV 11), Chengman (ST 20).

Weishu (BL 21), Youmen (KI 21), Liangmen (ST 21), Jinsuo (GV 18), Huaroumen (ST 24), Pishu (BL 20).

1) Shangwan (CV 13)

Location:On the midline of the abdomen, 5 cun above the umbilicus.

Function:To regulate the circulation of qi.

2) Zhongwan (CV 12)

Loction:On the midline of the abdomen, 4 cun above the umbilicus.

Function:To regulate the circulation of qi, harmonize the stomach functions, reduce the upward perversion of qi and eliminate damp.

3) Xiawan(CV 10)

Location:On the midline of the abdomen, 2 cun above the umbilicus.

Function: To regulate the circulation of qi and harmonize the Middle Energizer.

4) Burong (ST 19)

Location: 6 cun above the umbilicus and 2 cun lateral to Juque (CV 14), at the lower border of the region being adhere to the 8th rib.

Function: To regulate the stomach qi.

5) Taiyi (ST 23)

Location: 2 cun above the umbilicus, 2 cun lateral to Xiawan (CV 10).

Function: To calm down the mind and eliminate pain.

6) Zhangmen (LR 13)

Location: At the anterior end of the 11th rib, on the axillary midline.

Function: To regulate the liver qi, harmonize the stomach and strengthen the spleen.

7) Taibai (SP 3)

Location: Posterior and inferior to the head of the 1st metatarsal bone, in the depression at the junction of the red and white skin.

Function: To stop pain and promote digestion.

8) Zhongting (CV 16)

Location: On the midline of the sternum, at the level with the 5th intercostal space.

Function: To promote circulation in the meridian and collateral.

9) Yishe (BL 49)

Location: Inferior and lateral to the lower border of the spinous process of the 11th thoracic vertebra, 3 cun lateral to Governor Vessle.

Function: To regulate the functions of the spleen and stomach.

10) Juque (CV 14)

Location: On the midline of the abdomen, 6 cun above the umbilicus.

Function: To descend the upward perversion of

Zang qi.

11) Neiguan (PC 6)

Location: On the flexion side of the forearm, 2 cun posterior to the transverse crease of the wrist, between the tendons of m. palmaris longus and m. flexor radialis.

Function: To harmonize the Middle Energizer, stop pain, relax the chest, descend qi and calm down the mind.

12) Gongsun (SP 4)

Location: 1 cun above the digital joint of the big toe, on the medial aspect of the foot, and anterior and inferior to the base of the 1st metatarsal bone.

Function:To activate the circulation of blood, remove stagnation, strengthen the spleen and eliminate damp.

13) Quze (PC 3)

Location: In the centre of the transverse cubital crease, at the ulnar side of the tendon of m. biceps brachi.

Function: To ease the fright and eliminate pain.

14) Hegu (LI 4)

Location: On the dorsum of the hand, between the 1st and 2nd metacarpal bones, approximately in the middle of the 2nd metacarpal bone on the radial side.

Function: To disperse wind, eliminate the exterior syndromes, promote the circulation of qi and blood in the meridian and collateral and stop pain.

15) Guanmen (ST 22)

Location: 3 cun above the umbilicus and 2 cun lateral to Conception Vessel, 1 cun below Liang-men (ST 21).

Function: To regulate the functions of the spleen and stomach.

16) Zusanli (ST 36)

Location: 3 cun below the lower border of the patella and one finger-breadth lateral to the anterior crest of the tibia.

Function: To regulate the functions of the spleen and stomach, calm down the mind, stop pain and regulate and tonify qi and blood.

17) Jianshi (PC 5)

Location: On the flexion aspect of the forearm, 3 cun above the transverse crease of the wrist, between the tendons of m. palmaris longus and m. flexor carpi radials.

Function: To promote circulation in the meridian and collateral and calm down the mind.

18) Fuai (SP 16)

Location: Proximal to the 8th rib, 3 cun above Daheng (SP 15). On the muscular region of the lateral m. obliquus internus abdominis and transverse muscle of abdomen.

Function: To strengthen the spleen, harmonize the Middle Energizer, promote circulation in the meridian and collateral and mainly treat indigestion.

19) Lingxu (KI 24)

Location: 2 cun lateral to the anterior midline, in the 3rd intercostal space.

Function: To benefit the kidney, reduce the upward perversion of qi and mainly treat indigestion.

20) Jianli (CV 11)

Location: On the midline of the abdomen, 1 cun above the umbilicus.

Function: To regulate qi and harmonize the Middle Energizer.

21) Chengman (ST 20)

Location: 5 cun above the umbilicus and 2 cun lateral to the anterior midline, 1 cun below Burong (ST 19).

Function: To harmonize the stomach, stop pain, regulate qi and benefit the Middle Energizer.

22) Weishu (BL 21)

Location:1.5 cun lateral to the lower border of the spinous process of the 12th thoracic vertebra.

Function: To regulate the stomach qi.

23) Youmen (KI 21)

Location: 6 cun above the umbilicus and 0.5 cun lateral to the midline of the abdomen.

Function: To regulate the stomach qi.

24) Liangmen (ST 21)

Location: 4 cun above the umbilicus and 2 cun lateral to the anterior midline.

Function: To regulate the stomach qi, remove the accumulation of food and stagnation.

25) Jinsuo (GV 8)

Location: Below the spinous process of the 9th thoracic vertebra.

Function: To descend the upward perversion of qi, harmonize the functions of the stomach, disperse wind and open the orifice.

26) Huaroumen (ST 24)

Location: 1 cun above the umbilicus, 2 cun lateral to the midline of the abdomen.

Function:To regulate the function of the spleen and stomach and promote circultion in the meridian and collateral.

27) Pishu (BL 20)

Location: 1.5 cun lateral to the lower border of the spinous process of the 11th thoracic vertebra.

Function: To regulate the functions of the spleen and stomach.

24. Enteritis

Tianshu (ST 25), Gongsun (SP 4), Sanyinjiao (SP 6), Yinjiao (CV 7), Sanjiaoshu (BL 22), Xiajuxu (ST 39), Shangjuxu (ST 37), Dashangshu (BL 25), Xiaochangshu (BL 27), Shanglian (LI 9), Taibai (SP 3), Zhonglushu (BL 29), Changqiang (GV 1), Shuifen (CV 9), Hegu (LI 4), Guanyuanshu (BL 26), Guanyuan (CV 4), Guanmen (ST 22), Yanggang (BL 48), Zusanli (ST 36), Jianli (CV 11), Chengman (ST 20), Fuliu (KI 7), Shenque (CV 8), Youmen (KI 21), Jizhong (GV 6), Shangqu (KI 17) Wenliu (LI 7).

1) Tianshu (ST 25)

Locaiton: 2 cun lateral to the umbilicus.

Function: To regulate qi in the Middle Energizer.

2) Gongsun (SP 4)

Location: 1 cun posterior to the medial aspect of the digital joint of the big toe, at the anterior inferior to the base of the 1st metatarsal bone.

Function: To activate the circulation of blood, remove stagnation, strengthen the spleen functions to eliminate damp.

3) Sanyinjiao (SP 6)

Location: 3 cun directly above the tip of the medial malleolus, on the posterior border of the medial aspect of the tibia.

Function: To strengthen the spleen functions to resolve damp, smooth the liver qi, benefit the kidney functions, nourish yin and moisten dryness, benefit defecation to stop diarrhea.

4) Yinjiao (CV 7)

Location: On the midline of the abdomen, 1 cun below the umbilicus.

Function: To promote circulation in the meridian and collateral and stop pain.

5) Sanjiaoshu (BL 22)

Location: 1.5 cun lateral to the lower border of the spinous process of the 1st lumbar vertebra.

Function: To remove the stagnation of qi from the Triple Energizers.

6) Xiajuxu (ST 39)

Location: 3 cun below Shangjuxu (ST 37), one finger-breadth lateral to the anterior crest of the tibia.

Function: To calm down the mind and stop pain.

7) Shangjuxu (ST 37)

Location: 6 cun below the lower border of the

patella, one finger-breadth lateral to the anterior crest of the tibia.

Function: To promote circulation in the meridian and collateral, tonify qi and benefit the Middle Energizer.

8) Dachangshu (BL 25)

Location: 1.5 cun lateral to the lower border of the spinous process of the 4th lumbar vertebra, at the level with the upper border of the iliac crest.

Function: To regulate qi and stop pain.

9) Xiaochangshu (BL 27)

Location: 1.5 cun lateral to Governor Vessel, at the level with the 1st posterior sacral foramen, in the depression between the medial border of the posterior superior iliac spine and the sacrum.

Function: To regulate the digestive tract.

10) Shanglian (LI 9)

Location: 3 cun below Quchi (LI 11).

Function: To promote circulation in the meridian and collateral.

11) Taibai (SP 3)

Location: Proximal and inferior to the head of the 1st metatarsal bone, at the junction of the red and white skin.

Function: To stop pain and remove the accumulation of food.

12) Zhonglushu (BL 29)

Location: 1.5 cun lateral to Governor Vessel, at the level with the 3rd posterior sacral foramen.

Function: To tonify the kidney functions and strengthen the lumbus.

13) Changqiang (GV 1)

Location: Midway between the tip of the coccyx and the anus.

Function: To promote the circulation of qi and blood in Conception and Governor Vessels, strengthen yang qi and regulate the functions of Zang-fu organs.

14) Shuifeng (CV 9)

Location: On the midline of the abdomen, 1 cun above the umbilicus.

Function: To remove the accumulation of food, benefit water metabolism, and regulate the functions of the spleen and stomach.

15) Hegu (LI 4)

Location: On the dorsum of the hand, between the 1st and 2nd metacarpal bones, appoximately in the middle of the 2nd metacarpal bone on the radial side.

Function: To disperse wind, eliminate the exterior syndromes, promote the circulation of qi and blood in the meridian and collateral and stop pain.

16) Guanyuanshu (BL 26)

Location: 1.5 cun lateral to the lower border of the spinous process of the 5th lumbar vertebra.

Function: To strengthen the lumbus and the kidney functions.

17) Guanyuan (CV 4)

Location: On the midline of the umbilicus, 3 cun below the umbilicus.

Function: To strengthen the body resistance and the kidney functions, regulate qi and rescue yang.

18) Guanmen (ST 22)

Location: 3 cun above the umbilicus, 2 cun lateral to the anterior midline, 1 cun below Liangmen (ST 21).

Function: To regulate the functions of the spleen and stomach.

19) Yanggang (BL 48)

Location: 3 cun lateral to the lower border of the spinous process of the 10th thoracic vertebra.

Function: To smooth the liver qi, remove stagnation, clear away heat and remove toxin.

20) Zusanli (ST 36)

Location: 3 cun below the lower border of the patella, one finger-breadth lateral to the anterior crest of the tibia, in m. tibialis anterior.

Function: To regulate the functions of the spleen and stomach, tonify qi and blood, calm down the mind, stop pain and regulate the circulation of qi and blood.

21) Jianli (CV 11)

Location: On the midline of the abdomen, 1 cun above the umbilicus.

Function: To regulate qi and harmonize the Middle Energizer.

22) Chengman (ST 20)

Location: 5 cun above the umbilicus, 2 cun lateral to the anterior midline, 1 cun below Burong (ST 19).

Function: To regulate qi, benefit the Middle Energizer, harmonize the functions of the stomach and stop pain.

23) Fuliu (KI 7)

Location: In the depression 2 cun above the medial malleolus.

Function: To strengthen yang, eliminate the exterior syndromes, benefit the kidney functions and reduce edema.

24) Shenque (CV 8)

Location: In the centre of the umbilicus.

Function: To regulate the functions of the

spleen and stomach.

25) Youmen (KI 21)

Location: 6 cun above the umbilicus, 0.5 cun lateral to the midline of the abdomen.

Function: To regulate qi activity and stop pain.

26) Jizhong (GV 6)

Location: Below the spinous process of the 11th thoracic vertebra.

Function: To elevate yang, benefit qi, disperse wind and eliminate the exterior syndromes.

27) Shangqu (KI 17)

Location: 2 cun above the umbilicus and 0.5 cun lateral to the anterior midline.

Function: To nourish yin, benefit the kidney functions and disperse qi.

28) Wenliu (LI 7)

Location: On the radial side of the forearm, on the line joining Yangxi (LI 5) and Quchi (LI 11), 5 cun above Yangxi (LI 5).

Function: To eliminate pain and promote circulation in the meridian and collateral.

25. Colitis

Guanmen (ST 22), Guanyuan (CV 4), Yanggang (BL 48), Sanyinjiao (SP 6).

1) Guanmen (ST 22)

Location: 3 cun above the umbilicus and 2 cun lateral to the anterior midline, 1 cun below Liangmen (ST 21).

Function: To regulate the functions of the spleen and stomach.

2) Guanyuan (CV 4)

Location: 3 cun below the umbilicus, on the midline of the abdomen.

Function: To strengthen the body resistance, consolidate the kidney functions, regulate qi and rescue yang.

3) Yanggang (BL 48)

Location: 3 cun lateral to the lower border of the spinous process of the 10th thoracic vertebra.

Function: To smooth the liver qi,remove stagnation, clear away heat and remove toxin.

4) Sanyinjiao (SP 6)

Location: 3 cun directly above the tip of the medial malleolus, on the posterior border of the tibia.

Function: To strengthen the spleen functions to resolve damp, smooth the liver qi,benefit the kidney functions, nourish yin to moisten dryness, benefit defecation to stop diarrhea.

26.Cholecystitis.

Yinlingquan(SP 9), Junliao (GB 29), Danshu-

(BL 19), Dannang(Ex-LE6).

1) Yinlingquan(SP 9).

Location:Below the knee, on the medial aspect of the leg, in the depression below the medial condyle of the tibia.

Function: To resolve damp, remove stagnation, benefit the Lower Energizer and urination.

2) Juliao(GB 29)

Location: In the depression of the midpoint between the anterosuperior iliac spine and the great trochanter.

Function: To promote circulation in the meridian and collateral, expel wind and open the orifice.

3) Ganshu(BL 19)

Location: 1.5 cun lateral to the lower border of the spinous process of the 10th thoracic vertebra.

Function: To expel wind and benefit the gallbladder.

4) Gannang (Ex-LE 6).

Location: 1.5 cun anterior to the head of the fibula.

Function: To reduce inflammation and stop pain.

27.Constipation.

Dachangshu(BL 25), Kongzui(LU 6), Shiguan(KI 18), Siman(KI 14), Chengshan(BL 57), Zhibian(BL 54), Shangqu(KI 17), Hunmen(BL 47), Sanyinjiao(SP 6), Wushu(GB 27), Pan-gguangshu(BL 28), Shangjuxu(ST 37), Fenglong(ST 40), Taibai(SP 3), Hegu(LI 4), Yindu (KI 19), Chengfu(BL 36), Youmen(KI 21), Fuxi(BL 38), Huangmen(BL 51).

1) Dachangshu(BL 25)

Location: 1.5 cun lateral to the lower border of the spinous process of the 4th lumbar vertebra, at the level with the upper border of the iliac crest.

Function: To regulate qi and stop pain.

2) Kongzui (LU 6)

Location: On the line joining Chize (LU 5) and Taiyuan (LU 9), 5 cun below Chize (LU 5) and 7 cun above Taiyuan (LU 9).

Function: To clear away heat and ease pain.

3) Shiguan (KI 18)

Location: 3 cun above the umbilicus and 0.5 cun lateral to the anterior midline.

Function: To nourish yin, benefit the kidney functions, regulate qi circulation to stop pain.

4) Siman (KI 14)

Location: 2 cun below the umbilicus and 1.5 cun lateral to the anterior midline.

Function: To nourish yin and benefit the

kidney functions.

5) Chengshan (BL 57)

Location: On the posterior aspect of the leg, directly below the belly of m. gastrocnemius.

Function: To activate the circulation of blood to remove blood stasis and relieve spasm.

6) Zhibian (BL 54)

Location: 3 cun lateral to the lower border of the spinous process of the 4th sacral vertebra.

Function: To promote the circulation of qi in the meridian and collateral and harmonize the Middle Energizer.

7) Shangqu (KI 17)

Location: 2 cun above the umbilicus and 0.5 cun lateral to the anterior midline.

Function: To nourish yin, benefit the kidney functions and disperse qi.

8) Hunmen (BL 47)

Location: 3 cun lateral to the lower border of the spinous process of the 9th thoracic vertebra.

Function: To smooth the liver qi, benefit the gallbladder functions and promote the circulation of the meridian and collateral.

9) Sanyinjiao (SP 6)

Location: 3 cun directly above the tip of the medial malleolus, on the posterior border of the tibia.

Function: To strengthen the spleen functions to resolve damp, smooth the liver qi, benefit the kidney functions, nourish yin to moisten dryness, benefit defecation to stop diarrhea.

10) Wushu (GB 27)

Location: On the lateral side of the abdomen, in the front of the anterosuperior iliac spine, 3 cun below the umbilicus.

Function: To disperse wind and promote circulation in the meridian and collateral.

11) Pangguangshu (BL 28)

Location: 1.5 cun lateral to the lower border of the 2nd posterior sacral foramen, in the depression between the medial border of the posterior superior iliac spine and the sacrum.

Function: To reduce inflammation and benefit urination.

12) Shangjuxu (ST 37)

Location: 6 cun below the lower boder of the patella, one finger-breadth lateral to the anterior crest of the tibia.

Function: To tonify qi, benefit the Middle Energizer and promote circulation in the meridian and collateral.

13)Fenglong (ST 40)

Location: 8 cun anterior-superior above the external malledus, midway between the lower border of the patella and the external malleolus.

Function: To conduct yang flowing upward and smooth the circulation of qi.

14) Taibai (SP 3)

Location: Proximal and inferior to the head of the 1st metatarsal bone, at the junction of the red and white skin.

Function: To stop pain and reduce the accumulation of food.

15) Hegu (LI 4)

Location: On the dorsum of the hand, between the 1st and 2nd metacarpal bones, approximately in the middle of the 2nd metacarpal bone on the radial side.

Function: To disperse wind, eliminate the exterior syndromes, promote the circulation of qi and blood in the meridian and collateral and stop pain.

16) Yindu (KI 19)

Location: 4 cun above the umbilicus and 0.5 cun lateral to the anterior midline.

Function: To nourish yin, benefit the kidney functions, open the orifice and regain the consciousness.

17) Chengfu (BL 36)

Location: In the middle of the transverse gluteal fold. To locate the point in prone position.

Function: To strengthen the body resistance, eliminate the pathogenic factors, relax tendons and promote circulation in the meridian and collateral.

18) Yiumen(KI 21)

Location: 6 cun above the umbilicus,0.5 cun lateral to the midline of the abdomen.

Function: To regulate the stomach qi.

19) Fuxi(BL 38)

Location: 1 cun above Weiyang(BL 39), on the medial side of the tendon of m.biceps femonis.

Function: To expel wind and promote the circulation in the meridian and collateral.

20) Huangmen(BL 51)

Location: 3 cun lateral to the lower border of the spinous process of the 1st lumbar vertebra (Below the 13th vertebra).

Function: To promote circulation in the meridian and collateral.

28. Urination Disturbance

Shimen (CV 5), Pangguangshu (BL 28), Dachangshu (BL 25), Diji (SP 8), Ququan (LR 8), Yanglingquan (GB 34), Yinlingquan (SP 9), Zhishi (BL 52), Henggu (KI 11), Ligou (LR 5), Xingjian

(LR 2), Huiyin (CV 1), Chengfu (BL 36), Laogong (PC 8).

1) Shimen (CV 5)

Location: 2 cun below the umbilicus, on the midline of the abdomen.

Function: To balance yin and yang, benefit qi and blood.

2) Pangguangshu (BL 28)

Location: 1.5 cun lateral to the 2nd posterior sacral foramen. In the depression between the lower border of the posterior-superior iliac spine and the sacrum.

Function: To reduce inflammation and benefit urination.

3) Dachangshu (BL 25)

Location: 1.5 cun lateral to the lower border of the spinous process of the 4th lumbar vertebra, at the level with the upper border of the iliac crest.

Function: To regulate qi and stop pain.

4) Diji (SP 8)

Location: 3 cun below Yinlingquan (SP 9), on the line joining the tip of the medial malleolus and Yinlingquan (SP 9).

Function: To promote circulation in the meridian and collateral, strengthen the spleen functions to regulate qi circulation.

5) Ququan (LR 8)

Location: When the knee is flexed, the point is at the medial end of the transverse popliteal crease, posterior to the medial epicondyle of the tibia, in the depression of the end of the femur.

Function: To promote circulation in the meridian and collateral and smooth the liver qi.

6) Yanglingquan (GB 34)

Location: Lateral and inferior to the knee joint, in the depression anterior and inferior to the head of the fibula.

Function: To promote circulation in the meridian and collateral, eliminate damp and heat, smooth the liver qi and benefit the gallbladder functions.

7) Yinlingquan (SP 9)

Location: On the lower border of the medial condyle of the tibia, in the depression on the medial border of the tibia.

Function: To resolve damp, benefit the Lower Energizer and urination.

8) Zhishi (BL 52)

Location: 3 cun lateral to the lower border of the spinous process of the 2nd lumbar vertebra.

Function: To strengthen the lumbus and kidney functions.

9) Henggu (KI 11)

Location: 5 cun below the umbilicus and 0.5 cun lateral to the anterior midline.

Function: To nourish yin, benefit the kidney functions and strengthen the lumbus and knees.

10) Ligou (LR 5)

Location: 5 cun above the tip of the medial malleolus, in the centre of the medial aspect of the tibia.

Function: To smooth the liver qi and promote the circulation of blood in the meridian.

11) Xingjian (LR 2)

Location: On the dorsum of the foot between the 1st and 2nd toes, in the depression about 0.5 cun proximal to the margin of the web.

Function: To promote circulation in the meridian and collateral and smooth the liver qi.

12) Huiyin (CV 1)

Location: Between the anus and the root of the scrotum in males and between the anus and the posterior labial commissure in females.

Function: To regulate menstruation, remove stagnation and benefit urination.

13) Chengfu (BL 36)

Location: In the middle of the transverse gluteal fold. To locate the point in prone position.

Function: To strengthen the body resistane, eliminate the pathogenic factors, relax the tendons and promote circulation in the meridian and collateral.

14) Laogong (PC 8)

Location: On the transverse crease of the palm, between the 2nd and 3rd metacarpal bones. When the fist is clenched, the point is just below the tip of the middle finger.

Function: To nourish yin and calm down the mind.

29. Eye Disorders

Yuyao (Ex-HN4), Guangming (GB 37), Jingming (BL 1), Zanzhu (BL 2), Yangbai (GB 14), Tongziliao (GB 1), Zhongzu (TE 3), Fengchi (GB 20), Sizhukong (TE 23), Yuzhen (BL 9), Waiguan (TE 5), Dahe (KI 12), Shangxing (GV 23), Tianfu (LU 3), Shaoze (SI 1), Muchuang (GB 16), Sibai (ST 2), Toulingqi (GB 15), Touqiaoyin (GB 11),Touwei (ST 8), Zulinqi (GB 41), Ganshu (BL 18), Yanglao (SI 6), Tongtian (BL 7), Yinbai (SP 1), Jiexi (ST 41), Zhaohai (KI 6), Qiaojian (GV 18).

1) Yuyao (Ex-HN 4).

Location: At the midpoint of the eyebrow.

Function: To brighten the eyes,clear up the mind, expel wind and clear away heat.

2) Guangming(GB 37)

Location: 5 cun directly above the tip of the external malleolus, on the anterior border of the fibula, between m. extensor digitorum longus and m. peronaeus breais.

Function:To clear up the mind,brighten the eyes remove, stagnation and clear away heat.

3) Jingming (BL 1)

Location: In the depression superior to the inner canthus.

Function: To brighten the eyes,clear up the mind and treat various eye disorders.

4) Zanzhu(BL 2)

Location: In the depression on the medial extremity of the eyebrow, just above Jingming (BL 1).

Function: To disperse wind,brighten the eyes, clear up the mind and stop pain.

5) Yangbai (GB 14)

Location: on the forehead, 1 cun directly above the midpoint of the eyebrow. About at the junction of the upper 2/3 and the lower 1/3 of the line joining the anterior of the eyebrow, directly above the pupil when the eyes staring forward.

Function: To expel wind and ease pain.

6) Tongziliao (GB 1)

Location: 0.5 cun lateral to the outer canthus, on the lateral side of the orbit.

Function: To clear up the mind, brighten the eyes,dispel wind and clear away heat.

7) Zhongzu (TE 3)

Location: On the dorsum of the hand between the 4th and 5th metacarpal bones, in the depression proximal to the metacarpophalangeal joint.

Function: To expel wind, clear away heat, open the orifice and benefit the brain.

8) Fengchi (GB 20)

Location: In the depression between the upper portion of m. sternocleidomastoideus and m.trapezius, below the occiput.

Function: To expel wind, clear away heat and promote circulation in the meridian and callateral,

9) Sizhukong (TE 23)

Location: In the depression at the lateral end of the eyebrow.

Function: To expel wind, clear away heat, open the orifice and benefit the brain.

10) Yuzhen (BL 9)

Location: 1.3 cun lateral to Naohu (GV 17), on the lateral side of the superior border of the external occipital protuberance.

Function: To ease pain and calm down the

mind .

11) Waiguan (TE 5)

Location: 2 cun above the transverse crease of the wrist, on the dorsal aspect of the forearm, between the radius and ulna.

Funchion: To eliminate the exterior syndromes, clear away the heat and promote circulation in the meridian and collateral.

12) Dahe (KI 12)

Location: 4 cun below the umbilicus and 0.5 cun lateral to the anterior midline.

Function: To nourish yin and benefit the kidney functions.

13) Shangxing (GV 23)

Location: 1 cun within the anterior hairline,4 cun anterior to Baihui(GV 20).

Function: To clear the mind and brighten the eyes.

14) Tianfu (LU 3)

Location: On the medial aspect of the arm. 3 cun below the end of axillary fold, on the radial side of m. biceps brschii.

Function: To promote circulation in the meridian and collateral.

15) Shaoze (SI 1)

Location: On the ulnar side of the little finger,

about 0.1 cun posterior to the corner of the nail.

Function: To clear away heat and moisten dryness.

16) Muchuang (GB 16)

Location: 1.5 cun posterior to Toulinqi(GB 15) , on the line joining Toulinqi (GB 15) and Fengchi (GB 20).

Function: To clear up the mind, brighten the eyes, expel wind, clear away heat and treat cataract, glaucoma, etc.

17) Sibai (ST 2)

Location: With the eyes looking straight forward, directly below the pupil, in the depression at the infraorbital foramen.

Function: To clear away heat and expel wind.

18) Touqiaoyin (GB 11)

Location: Posterior and superior to the mastoid process, behind the ear.

Function: To clear up the mind and open the orifice.

19) Toulinqi (GB 15)

Location: With the eyes looking straight forward, 0.5 cun within the hairline directly above the pupil, midway between Shenting (GV 24) and Touwei (ST 8).

Function: To calm down the mind and promote

circulation in the meridian and collateral.

20) Touwei (ST 8)

Location: 0.5 cun within the anterior hairline at the corner of the forehead, 4.5 cun lateral to Shenting (GV 24).

Function: To eliminate heat and stop pain.

21) Zulinqi (GB 41)

Location: In the depression distal to the junction of the 4th and 5th metatarsel bones.

Function: To regulate the liver functions and brigthen the eyes.

22) Ganshu (BL 18)

Location: 1.5 cun lateral to the lower border of the spinous process of the 9th thoracic vertebra.

Function: To effect resuscitation and improve vision.

23) Yanglao (SI 6)

Location: Dorsal to the head of the ulna. When the palm faces the chest, the point is in the bony clef on the radial side of the styloid process of the ulna.

Function: To smooth the tendons and promote vision.

24) Tongtian (BL 7)

Location: 1.5 cun posterior to Chengguang (BL 6), anterior to Baihui (GV 20).

Function: to promote qi of Foot Taiyang.

25) YinBai (SP 1)

Location: On the medial side of the big toe, about 0.1 cun posterior to the corner of the nail.

Function: To nourish qi and blood.

26) Jiexi (ST 41)

Location: In the depression of midpoint of the transverse crease at the junction of the dorsum of foot and leg.

Function: To clear heat from up jiao and promote circulation of meridian and collaterals.

27) Zhaohai (KI 6)

Location: In the depression and one cun below the medial malleolus.

Function: To activate blood and stop pain, to calm the patient.

28) Qiangjian (GV 18)

Location: In the depression between parietal bone and occipital bone, 1.5 cun posterior to Houding (GV 19)

Function: To relax the wind and to promote the collaterals.

30. Desease of the ear

Tinggong (SI 19), Tinghui (GV 2), Zulingi (GV41), Zuqiaoyin (GV 44), Yifeng (TE 17), Sanyangluo (TE 8), Xiaguan (ST 7), Yemen (TE2), Zhigou

(TE 6), Tianjing (TE 10), Tianrong (SI 17) Zhongzhu (TE 3), Sidu (TE9), Waiguan (TE 5), TouqiaoYin (GV 11), Ermen (TE 21), Hegu (LI 4), Yangchi (TE4), Yangxi (LI 5), Shenshu (BL 23), Jianjing (GB 21), Jianzhen (TE 9), Pianli (LI 6).

1) Tinggong:(SI 19)

Location: Between the tragus and mandibular joint, where a depression is fonmed wherr the mouth is slightly open.

Function: To clear the fire and calm the patient.

2) Tinghui: (GB 2)

Location: Anterior to the intertragic notch, at the posterior border of the condyloid process of the mandible. There is a depression when the mouth is opened.

Function: To promote circulation of meridian and collaterals, to eliminate wind and effect resuscitation.

3) Zulinqi: (GB 41)

Location: In the depression distal to the junction of the 4th and 5th metatarsal bones.

Fuction: To regulate liver qi and clear vision.

4) Zuqiaoyin (GB 44)

Location: On the lateral side of the 4th toe, about 0.1 cun posterior to the corner of the nail.

Function: To clear fire from upper jiao.

5)Yifeng (TE 17)

Location: Posterior to the lobule of the ear, between the mandible and mastoid process.

Function: To promote circulation of the meridian and collaterals, and to clear the hearing.

6) Sanyangluo (TE 8)

Location: Posterior to the wrist of the forearm, between the radius and ulna.

Function: To clear the hearing and to eliminate wind and heat.

7) Xiaguan (ST 7)

Location: In the depression at the lower border of the zygomatic arch anterior to the condyloid process of the mandible when the mouth is closed.

Function: To clear heat and stop pain.

8) Yemen (TE 2)

Location: Proximal to the margin of the web between the ring and small fingers. The point is located with clenched fist.

Function: Brighteen the eyes binefity brein.

9) Zhigou (TE 6)

Location: 3 cun posterior to the lateral side of forearm, between the ulna and radius.

Function: To promote circulation of the meridian and collaterals.

10) Tianjing (TE 10)

Location: When the elbow is flexed, the point is in the depression about 1 cun superior to the olecranon.

Function: To effect resuscitation and brighteen the eyes.

11) Tianrong (SI 17)

Location: Posterior to the angle of mandible, in the depreesion on the anterior border of m. sternocleidomastoideus.

Function: To eliminate heat and relax the toxin.

12) Zhongzhu (TE 3)

Location: Between the 4th and 5th metacarpl bones, in the depression proximal to the metacarpoph alangeal joint.

Function: To relive the wind and heat, and effect resuscitation and brighteen eyes.

13) Sidu (TE 9)

Location: Posterior to the forearm, 5 cun below the elbow. at anterior border of the unlna.

Function: To eliminate wind and stop pain, to promote circulation of the meridian and collatarals.

14) Waiguan: (TE 5)

Location: Between the radius and ulna, 2 cun

posterior to the transverse crease of the wrist and forearm.

Function: To promote circulation of the meridian and collaterals, to eliminate exterior heat.

15) Touqiaoyin: (GB 11)

Location: Posterior and superior to the mostoid process.

Function: To effect resuscitation.

16) Ermen: (TE 21)

Location: In the depression anterior to the supratragic notch, The point is located when the mouth is opened.

Function: To clear hearing.

17) Hegu (LI 4)

Location: Between the 1st and 2nd metacarpal bones, approximately in the middle of the 2nd metacarpal bones, approximately in the middle of the 2nd metacarpal bone on the radial side.

Function: To eliminate wind from Biao exterior syndrome and promote circulation of meridian and colleterals. to effect resuscitation and stop pain. to activate qi and blood.

18) Yangchi:(TE 4)

Location: At the junction of the ulna and carpal bones, in the depression lateral to the tendon of m. extensor digitorum communis.

Function: To clear vision and hearing and promote circulation of the joints.

19) Yangxi: (LI 5)

Location: On the ralial side of the wrist. When the thumb is tilted upward, it is in he depression between the tendons of m. extensor pollicis logus and brevis.

Function: To clear wind heat, to active qi and blood.

20) Shenshu (BL 23)

Location: 1.5 cun lateral to the lower border of the spinous process of the 2nd lumber vertebra.

Function: To tonife the kidney and treat deafness and tinnitus.

21) Jianjing (GB 21)

Location: Midway between Dazhui (DU 14) and the acromion.

Function: To promote circulation of the meridian and collaterals, and to eliminate wind and stop pain.

22) Jian zhen (SI 9)

Location: Posterior and inferior to the shoulder joint. When the arm is adducted, the point is 1 cun above the posterior end of of the axillary fold.

Function: To relax the tendons and smooth the collaterals.

23) Pianli (LI 6)

Location: 3 cun posterior to the wirst, on the radial side of the joint of the wrist, it is in the depression between the tendons of m. extensor pollicis longus and brevis.

Function: To activate the dispersing function of the lungus and brevis.

31. Desease of the Nose

Yingxiang (LI 20), Suliao (GV 25), Yintang (Ex-HN3), Shanxing (GV 24), Tianfu (LU 3), Tianzhu (BL 10), Juliao (ST3), Fengchi (GB 20), Toulinqi (GB 15), Yangbai (GB 14), Chengling (GB 18), Yuzhen (BL 9), Chengguang (BL 6).

1) Yingxia (LI 20)

Location: In the nasolabial groove, at the level of the midpoint of the lateral border of ala nasi.

Function To promote obstruction of nose.

2) Suliao (GV 25)

Location: On the tip of the nose.

Function: To eliminate heat and effect rasuscitation, to resolve phlegm.

3) Yintang (Ex-HN3)

Location: Midway between the medial ends of the two eyebrows.

Function: To eliminate heat and toxin and clear wind and regin consciousness.

4) Shangxing (GV 23)

Location: 1 cun within the anterior hairline, 4 cun anterior to Baihui (GV 20)

Function: To effect resuscitation and clear vision.

5) Tianfu (Lu 3)

Location: On the medial aspect of the upper arm, 3 cun below the end of the axillary fold, on the radial side of m. biceps brachii.

Function: To eliminate wind and promote circulation qi of meridian and collaterals.

6) Tianzhu (BL 10)

Location: 1.3 cun lateral to Yamen (GV 15) on the lateral side of m. trapezius.

Function: To clear mind and effect resuscitation.

7) Juliao (ST 3)

Location: At the level of the lower border of ala nasi.

Function: To promote circulation of the meridian and collaterals.

8) Fengchi (GB 20)

Location: In the posterior aspect of the neck, below the occipital bone, in the depression between the occipital bone, of m. sternacleidomastoideus. and m. trapezius.

Function: To clear wind and heat, and to promote circulation of meridian and collaterals, and to clear vision.

9) Toulinqi (GB 15)

Location: 0.5 cun within the hairline, midway between shenting (GB 24) and Touwei (ST 8)

Function: To calm the patient.

10) Yangbai (GB 14)

Location: On the forehead, 0.5 cun above the midpoint of the eyebrow, approximately at the junction of the upper two-thirds and lower third of the vertioal line drawn from the anterior hairline to the eyebrow.

Function: To eliminate wind and stop pain.

11) Chengling (GB 18)

Location 1.5 cun posterior to Muchuang (GB 18), on the line connecting Head-Linqi (GB 15) and Fengchi (GB 20)

Function: To eliminate wind and heat and to promote circulation of meridian and collaterals.

12) Yuzhen (BL 9)

Location: 1.3 cun lateral to Naohu (DU 17), On the lateral side of the superior border of the external occipital protuberance.

Function: To calm the patient and to stop pain.

13) Chengguang (BL 6)

Location: 1.5 cun posterion to Wuchu (BL 5), it is located on the top of the head.

Function: To effect nesuscitation and soothes mind.

32. Sore Throat

Shaoshang (LU 11). Lianquan (CV 23), Renying (ST 8), Tianzhu (BL 10), Tianding (BL 17), Tianrong (SI 17), Zhongzhu (TE 3), Neiting (ST 44), Qishe (ST 11), Kongzui (LU 6), Houxi (SI 3), Sanyanluo (TE 8), Zhigou (TE 6), Tiantu (CV 22), Fengfu (GV 16), Lidui (ST 45), Sidu (TE 9), Lieque (LU 7), Hegu (LI 4), Yangjiao (GB 35), Yuji (LU 10), Tongli (HT 5), Pianli (LI 6), Yemen (TE 2), Wenliu (LI 7), Qiguan.

1) Shaoshang (LU 11)

Location: On the radial side of the thumb, about 0.1 cun posterior to the corner of the nail.

Function: To stop cough and moisten the lung.

2) Lianquan (CV 23)

Location: Above the adam's apple, in the middle of the lower border of the tongue.

Function: To recapture yang and avert the collapeing state.

3) Renying (ST 9)

Location: 1.5 cun lateral to both sides of Adam's apple, on the anterior border of m. sternocleido-mastoideus.

Function: To promote circulation of meridians and eliminate wind

4) Tianzhu (BL 10)

Location: 1.3 cun lateral to Yamen (GV 15) on the lateral side of m. trapezius.

Function: To effect resuscitation and promote vision.

5) Tianding (LI 17)

Location: On the Posterior border of m. sternocleidomastoideus, 1 cun below Neck-Futu (LI 18).

Function: To eliminate edema and activate blood circulation.

6) Tiangrong (SI 17)

Location: Posterior to the angle of mandible, on the anterior border of m. sternocleidomastoideus.

Function: To clear heat and toxin.

7) Zhongzhu: (TE 3)

Location: The point is on the dorsum of hand between the 4th and 5th metacarpal bones in the depression proximal to the metacarpophalangeal joint.

Function: To eliminate wind heat and effect resuscitalion.

8) Neiting: (ST 44)

Location: Proximal to the web margin between the second and third toes. in the depression distal and lateral to the second metatarsodigital joint.

Function: To regulate qi and stop pain.

9) Qishe (ST 11)

Location: At the superior border of the sternal extremity of the clavicle, between the sternal head and clavicular head of m. sternocleidomastoideus.

Function: To activate stagnation of blood and regulate qi.

10) Kongzui: (LU 6)

Location: On the line joining Taiyuan (LU 9) and Chize (LU 5) 7 cun above the transverse crease of the wrist.

Function: To eliminate heat and stop pain. To stop asthma and cough.

11) Houxi (SI 3)

Location: When a loose fist is made, the point is on the ulnar side, proximal to the fifth metacarpophalangeal joint, at the end of the transverse crease and the junction of the red and white skin.

Function: Clearing away heat, eliminating wind, dredging the meridians and collaterals.

12) Sanyangluo (TE 8)

Location: 4 cun above the transverse crease of

the dorsum of wrist, between the radius and ulna.

Function: Eliminating wind and clearing away heat, promoting the ear function.

13) Zhigou (TE 6)

Location: 3 cun above the transverse crease of the dorsum of wrist, between the radius and ulna.

Function: Dredging the meridians and moving the blood in the collaterals, normalizing the function of gallbladder, descending the adverse flow of qi.

14) Tiantu (CV 22)

Location: In the centre of the suprasternal fossa.

Function: Descending Qi, promoting and relieving cough.

15) Fengfu (GV 16)

Location: 1 cun directly above the midpoint of the posterior hairline, directly below the external occipital protuberance, in the depression between m. trapezius of both sides.

Function: Eliminating pathogenic wind.

16) Lidui (ST 45)

Location: On the lateral side of the 2nd toe, 0.1 cun posterior to the corner of the nail.

Function: Suppressing pain and tranquilizing the mind.

17) Sidu (TE 9)

Location: On the lateral side of forearm, 5 cun below the olecranon, between the radius and ulna.

Function: Dispersing wind, suppressing pain and removing the obstruction from the meridians and collaterals.

18) Lieque (LU 7)

Location: Superior to the styloid process of the radius 1.5 cun above the transverse crease of the wrist. When the index fingers and thumbs of both hands are crossed with the index finger of one hand placed on the styloid process of the radius of the other, the point is in the depression right under the tip of the index finger.

Function: Removing the obstruction from the meridian and collateral, moistening the lung to stop cough.

19) Hegu (LI 4)

Location: On the dorsum of the hand, between the 1st and 2nd metacarpal bones, approximately in the middle of the 2nd metacarpal bone on the radial side.

Function: Eliminating wind, relieving symptoms of exterior syndromes, opening the meridians and the orifices, moving Qi and blood and removing obstruction from the collaterals to stop pain.

20) Yangjiao (GB 35)

Location: 7 cun above the tip of the external malleolus, on the posterior border of fibula.

Function: Dispersing the obstructive Qi, relieving convulsions.

21) Yuji (LU 10)

Location: On the radial aspect of the midpoint of the first metacarpal bone, on the junction of the red and white skin (i.e., the junction of the dorsum and palm of the hand)

Function: suppressing cough and asthma.

22) Tongli(H 5)

Location:When the palm faces upward, the point is on the radial side of the tendon of m. flexor carpi ulnaris, 1 cun above the transverse crease of the wrist.

Function: Tranquilizing the mind, opening the collaterals.

23) Pianli (LI 6)

Location: 3 cun above the dorsal aspect of the wrist, between the tendon of long extensor muscle of thumb and that of short extensor muscle of thumb.

Function: Activating lung's function and promoting dyuresis.

24) Yemen (TE 2)

Location: Proximal to the margin of the web between the ring and small fingers. The point is located with clenched fist.

Function: Promting the smooth flow of qi

25) Wenliu (LI 7)

Location: When a fist is made with the ulnar side downward and elbow flexed the point is 5cun above Yangxi (LI 5).

Function: Smoothing the circulation of-Qi and blood, relieving the sorenesss.

26) Xiguan (LR 7)

Location: Posterior and inferior to the medial condyle of the tibia, in the upper portion of the medial head of m. gastrocnemius, 1 cun posterior to Yinlingquan(SP 9).

Function: Eliminating wind and cold.

33.Hemiplegia

Shangjuxu (ST 37), Shanglian (LI 9), Fengshi (GB 31), Yanglingquan (GB 34), Huantiao (GB 30), Weizhong (BL 40), Jianjing (GB 21), Femur-Juliao (GB 29), Chengjiang (CV 24), Xuanzhong (GB 39),Yinbai(SP 1), Biguan(ST 31), Fengfu(GV 16), Yamen (GV 15)

1) Shangjuxu (ST 37)

Location: 6 cun below Dubi(ST 35), one finger-breadth from the anterior crest of the tibia.

Function: Promoting the flow of qi, reinforcing the qi of the spleen and stomach.

2) Shanglian (LI 9)

Location: 3 cun below Quchi (LI 11)

Function: Removing the obstruction from the meridians and collaterals.

3) Fengshi (GB 31)

Location: On the midline of the lateral aspect of the thigh, 7 cun above the transverse popliteal crease. When the patient is standing erect with the hands close to the sides, the point is where the tip of the middle finger touches.

Function: Dredging the meridians and collaterals, removing dampness and wind.

4) Yanglingquan (GB 34)

Location: In the depression anterior and inferior to the head of the fibula.

Function: Opening the meridians, moving the blood, clearing away heat and removing dampness.

5) Huantiao (GB 30)

Location: In the depression superior, posterior to the great trochanter.

Function: Dredging the meridians and collaterals, eliminating wind and cold, strengthening the waist and legs.

6) Weizhong (BL 40)

Location: Midpoint of the transverse crease of the popliteal fossa, between the tendons of m.biceps femoris and m. semitendinosus.

Function: Regulating the flow of qi, opening the meridian and moving the blood, removing summer heat.

7) Jianjing (GB 21)

Location: Midway between Dazhui (GV 14) and the acromion, at the highest point of the shoulder.

Function: Dredging the meridian and moving the blood, eliminating wind and relieving pain, relaxing the chest, promoting qi descending,

8) Femur-Juliao (GB 29)

Location:Midway between the anterosuperior iliac spine and the great trochanter.

Function: Dredging the meridian and activating blood circulation.

9) Chengjiang (CV 24)

Location:In the depression in the centre of the mentolabial groove.

Function: Eliminating wind,opening the collateral, relieving spasm and pain.

10) Xuanzhong (GB 39)

Location: 3 cun above the tip of the external malleolus, in the depression between the posterior border of the fibula and the tendons of m. peronaeus longus and brevis.

Function: Opening the meridian, moving the Qi and blood in the collaterals, eliminating wind and dampness.

11) Yinbai (SP 1)

Location: On the medial side of the big toe, about 0.1 cun posterior to the corner of the nail.

Function: Regulating blood replenishing spleen.

12) Biguan (ST 31)

Location: Directly below the anterior superior iliac spine, in the depression of the lateral side of m. sartorius when the thigh is flexed.

Function: Removing obstruction from the meridians and collaterals, moving qi and blood.

13) Fengfu (GV 16)

Location: Directly below the external occipital protuberance, in the depression between m. trapezius of both sides.

Function: Eliminating pathogenic wind.

14) Yamen (GV 15)

Location: At midpoint of the nape, 0.5 cun below Fengfu (GV 16) in the depression 0.5 cun within the hairline.

Function: Eliminating wind, easing the throat,

treating aphasia.

34. Dysmenorrhea and Irregular Menstruation

Diji(SP 8), Zhongji (CV 3), Qihai (CV 6), Dadun (LR 1), Tianshu (ST 25), Shimen (CV 5), Shiguan (KI 18) Guilai (ST 29), Siman (KI 14), Qugu (CV 2), Huiyin (CV 1), Guanyuan (CV 4), Yinlingquan (SP 9), Jingmen (GB 25), Daimai (GB 26) Yinbai (SP 1), Zhaohai (KI 6), Yaoshu (GV 2), Yaoyangguan (GV 3), Jimen (SP 11), Ligou (LR 5), Xuehai (SP 10), Sanyinjiao (SP 6), Qixue (KI 13), Baihuanshu (BL 30), Xingjian (LR 2), Shenshu (BL 23).

1) Diji (SP 8)

Location: 3 cun below the medial condyle of the tibia, on the line connecting Yinlingquan (SP 9) and the medial malleolus.

Function: Opening the meridian and activating the blood circulation in the collaterals, strengthening the spleen, and regulating the flow of qi.

2) Zhongji (CV 3)

Location: on the anterior midline, 4 cun below the umbilicus.

Function: Promoting Yang, harmonizing Yin, replenishing Qi and moving blood.

3) Qihai (CV 6)

Location: On the midline of the abdomen, 1.5 cun below the umbilicus.

Function: Reinforcing Qi, regulating blood, strengthening the spleen and kidney.

4) Dadun (LR 1)

Location:On the Lateral side of the dorsum of the terminal phalanx of great toe, between the lateral corner of the nail and interphalangeal joint.

Function: Regulating the meridian and suppressing pain, soothing the liver, regulating the flow of qi,

5) Tianshu (ST 25)

Location: 1 cun lateral to the centre of the umbilicus.

Function: Regulating the flow of Qi, normalizing the function of spleen and stomach.

6) Shimen (CV 5)

Location: On the midline of the abdomen, 1 cun below the umbilicus.

Function:Replenishing Qi and harmonizing the blood, strengthening yang,regulating Yin.

7) Shiguan (KI 18)

Location: 3 cun above the umbilicus, 0.5 cun lateral to the anterior midline.

Function: Regulating the flow of Qi, relieving pain, nourishing Yin, and replenishing kidney.

8) Guilai (ST 29)

Location: 4 cun below the umbilicus, I cun

lateral to the anterior midline.

Function:Regulating the flow of Qi,stopping pain.

9) Siman (KI 14)

Location: 2 cun below the umbilicus, 0.5 cun lateral to Shimen (Ren 5).

Function: Nourishing kidney yin.

10) Qugu (CV 2)

Location: On the midline of the abdomen, just above the symphysis pubis.

Function:Nourishing Yin, reinforcing Yang.

11) Huiyin (CV 1)

Location: In the centre of the perineum. It is between the anus and the scrotum in males and between the anus and posterior labial commissure in females,

Function: Regulating menstruation, normalizing leukorrhea.

12) Guanyuan (CV 4)

Location: On the midline of the abdomen,3 cun below the umbilicus.

Function: Regulating Qi, regaining Yang, reinforcing the kidney.

13) Yinlingquan (SP 9)

Location: On the lower border of the medial condyle of the tibia, in the depression between the posterior border of the tibia and m.gastrocnemius.

Funtion: Removing dampness, regulating menstruation, relieving pain, promoting urination, and smoothing the function of Lower Jiao.

14) Jingmen (GB 25)

Location: On the lateral side of the abdomen, on the lower border of the free end of the 12th rib.

Function: Regulating the water passage, relieving the fear and terror.

15) Daimai (GB 26)

Location: Directly below the free end of the 11th rid, level with the umbilicus.

Function: Regulating the flow of qi and the functions of spleen and stomach.

16) Yinbai (SP 1)

Location: On the medial side of the big toe, about 0.1 cun posterior to the corner of the nail.

Function:Benefiting the spleen, regulating the blood function.

17) Zhaohai (KI 6)

Location:In the depression directly below the medial malleolus.

Function: Moving the blood, relieving pain and calming down the mind.

18) Yaoshu (GV 2)

Location:In the hiatus of the sacrum.

Function:Strengthening the kidney and loins.

19) Yaoyangguan (GV 3)

Location:Below the spinous process of the 4th lumbar vertebra.

Function:Regulating qi and blood, reinforcing kidney and Yang Qi

20) Jimen (SP 11)

Location:On the medial side of the thigh, 8 cun above the patella.

Function:Reinforcing spleen and kidney.

21) Ligou (LR 5)

Location:5 cun above the tip of the medial malleolus, on the medial aspect and near the medial border of the tibia.

Function: Opening the meridian and moving the blood,soothing the liver and regulating the flow of qi.

22) Xuehai (SP 10)

Location:When the knee is flexed, the point is 2 cun above the mediosuperior border of the patella, on the bulge of the medial portion of m. quadriceps femoris.

Function:Regulating blood, relieving itching.

23) Sanyinjiao (SP 6)

Location: 3 cun directly above the tip of the medial malleolus,on the posterior border of the tibia, on the line drawn from the medial malleolus to Yinlingquan(SP 9).

Function:Strengthening the spleen, resolving dampness, nourishing Yin and moistening the dryness,soothing the liver and reinforcing the kidney, regulating the menstruation and treating uterine bleeding.

24) Qixue (KI 13)

Location:3 cun below the umbilicus, 0.5 cun lateral to the anterior midline.

Function:Regulating the flow of qi and blood.

25) Baihuanshu (BL 30)

Location:At level of the 4th posterior sacral foramen 1.5 cun lateral to the Governor Vessel.

Function:Strengthening the function of kidney, reinforcing the loins,

26) Xingjian (LR 2)

Location:Between the 1st and 2nd toe, proximal to the margin of the web.

Function:Removing the obstruction from the meridians and collaterals and moving the blood.

27) Shenshu (BL 23)

Location:1.5 cun lateral to the lower border of the spinous process of the 2nd lumbar vertebra.

Function:Strengthening the kidney and the low back.

35.Mastitis and Mastoplastia

Shanzhong (CV 17), Xiajuxu (ST 39).Guan-gming (GB 37), Huangmen (BL 51), Lingxu(KI 24), Jianjing (GB 21),Wuyi (ST 15), Diwuhui (GB 42)

1) Shanzhong (CV 17)

Location: On the midline of sternum,between the nipples, level with the 4th intercostal space,

Function: Regulating the flow of qi, descending the Qi, removing the fullness from the chest.

2) Xiajuxu (ST 39)

Location: 3 cun below Shangjuxu (ST 37) one finger-breath from the anterior crest of the tibia.

Function: To calm the patient and stop pain.

3) Guangming (GB 3)

Location: 5 cun directly above the tip of the external malleolus, on the anterior border of the fibula.

Function: To clear heat and stagnation of qi and blood.

4) Huangmen (BL 51)

Location: 3 cun lateral to the first lumbar vertebra, it is below the thirteenth vertebra.

Function: To relax the tendons and activate blood.

5) Lingxu (KI 24)

Location: In the third intercostal space, 2 cun

lateral to midline of the chest.

Function: To tonify the kidney qi.

6) Jianjing: (GB 21)

Location: Midway between Dazhui (GV 14) and acromin.

Function: To eliminate wind and stop pain. To relax the chest region and promote circulation of qi in meridian and collaterals.

7) Wuyi (ST 15)

Location: In the second intercostal space, 4 cun lateral to the midline of the chest.

Function: To clear heat and stop pain.

8) Diwuhui: (GB 42)

Location: Between the fourth and fifth metatarsal bones, on the medial border of the tendon of m. extensor digiti minimi of foot.

Function: To effect resuscitation and promote circulation of qi in meridian and collaterals.

36. The common points for health care

(1-2 points can be selected each time) Yongquan (KI 1), Zusanli (ST 36), Guanyuan (CV 4), Shenshu (BL 23), Yanglao (SI 6), Hegu (LI 4), Laogong (PC 8), Baihui (GV 20), Mingmen (GV 4), Taiyang (Ex-HN3), Guanyuanshu (BL 26).

1) Youngquan (KI 1)

Location: On the sole, in the depression when

the foot is in planter flexion.

Function: To promote circulation of qi in the meridian and collaterals. To nourish the liver, To eliminate wind and fire.

2) Zusanli (ST 36)

Location: 3 cun below Dubi (ST 35), one finger-breath from anterior crest of the tibia.

Function: To tonify qi and blood To regulate qi of spleen and stomach.

3) Guanyuan (CV 4)

Location: On the midine of the abdomen, 3 cun below the umbilicus.

Function: To regulate qi and restore yang.

4) Shenshu (BL 23)

Location: 1.5 cun lateral to Mingmen (GV 4) at the level of the second lumbar vertebra.

Function: To tonify the kidney and lumbus.

5) Yanglao: (SI 6)

Location: Dorsal to the head of the ulna. When the palm faces the chest, the point is in the bony cleft on the radial side of the styloid process of the ulna.

Function: To promote vision and relax the tendons.

6) Hegu:(LI 4)

Location: On the dorsum of the hand, between

the 1st and 2nd metacarpal bones.

Function: To eliminate wind and promote circulation of qi in meridian and collaterals. To activate qi and blood. To effect resuscitation.

7) Laogong: (PC 8)

Location: On the transverse creas of the palm, between the second and third metacarpal bones. When the fist is clenched, the point is just below the tip of the middle finger.

Function: To nourish yin and calm the patient

8) Baihui: (GV 20)

Location: On the midline of the head, 7 cun directly above the posterior hairline, approximately on the midpoint of the line connecting the apexes of the two auricles.

Function: To reduce wind and pacify the liver.

9) Mingmen (GV 4)

Location: Below the spinous process of the second lumbar vertebra.

Function: To tonify yang and qi of kidney, to promote lumbar vetebra, to calm the patient.

10) Taiyang: (EX-HN 5)

Location: In the depression about 1 cun posterior to the midpiont between the lateral end of the eyebrow and outer canthus.

Function: To eliminate wind and heat, to

promote circulation of Qi in meridian and collaterals. To promote vision.

11) Guanyuanshu (BL 26)

Location: 1.5 cun lateral to the Governor vessel, at the level of the lower border of the spinous process of the fifth lumbar vertebra.

Function: To strengthen the kidney.

Points of Lung Meridian, **LU.**
Shǒutàiyīn Fèijīng xué

LU 1	Zhōngfǔ	LU 7	Lièquē
LU 2	Yúnmén	LU 8	Jīngqú
LU 3	Tiānfǔ	LU 9	Tàiyuān
LU 4	Xiábái	LU 10	Yújì
LU 5	Chǐzé	LU 11	Shàoshāng
LU 6	Kǒngzuì		

Points of Large Intestine Meridian, **LI.**
Shǒuyángmíng Dàchángjīng xué

LI 1	Shāngyáng	LI 12	Zhǒuliáo
LI 2	Èrjiān	LI 13	Shǒuwǔlǐ
LI 3	Sānjiān	LI 14	Bìnào
LI 4	Hégǔ	LI 15	Jiānyú
LI 5	Yángxī	LI 16	Jùgǔ
LI 6	Piānlì	LI 17	Tiāndǐng
LI 7	Wēnliū	LI 18	Fútū
LI 8	Xiàlián	LI 19	Kǒuhéliáo *
LI 9	Shànglián		Héliáo§
LI 10	Shǒusānlǐ	LI 20	Yíngxiāng
LI 11	Qūchí		* § Either of these can be used.

Points of Stomach Meridian, **ST.**
Zúyángmíng Wèijīng xué

ST 1	Chéngqì	ST 24	Huáròumén
ST 2	Sìbái	ST 25	Tiānshū
ST 3	Jùliáo	ST 26	Wàilíng
ST 4	Dìcāng	ST 27	Dàjù
ST 5	Dàyíng	ST 28	Shuǐdào
ST 6	Jiáchē	ST 29	Gūilái
ST 7	Xiàguān	ST 30	Qìchōng
ST 8	Tóuwéi	ST 31	Bìguān
ST 9	Rényíng	ST 32	Fútù
ST 10	Shuǐtū	ST 33	Yīnshì
ST 11	Qìshè	ST 34	Liángqiū
ST 12	Quēpén	ST 35	Dúbí
ST 13	Qìhù	ST 36	Zúsǎnlǐ
ST 14	Kùfáng	ST 37	Shàngjùxū
ST 15	Wūyì	ST 38	Tiáokǒu
ST 16	Yīngchuāng	ST 39	Xiàjùxū
ST 17	Rǔzhōng	ST 40	Fēnglóng
ST 18	Rǔgēn	ST 41	Jiěxī
ST 19	Bùróng	ST 42	Chōngyáng
ST 20	Chéngmǎn	ST 43	Xiàngǔ
ST 21	Liángmén	ST 44	Nèitíng
ST 22	Guānmén	ST 45	Lìdùi
ST 23	Tàiyǐ		

Points of Spleen Meridian, **SP.**
Zútàiyīn Píjīng xué

SP 1	Yǐnbái	SP 12	Chōngmén
SP 2	Dàdū	SP 13	Fǔshè
SP 3	Tàibái	SP 14	Fùjié
SP 4	Gōngsūn	SP 15	Dàhéng
SP 5	Shāngqiū	SP 16	Fù'āi
SP 6	Sānyīnjiāo	SP 17	Shídòu
SP 7	Lǒugǔ	SP 18	Tiānxī
SP 8	Dìjī	SP 19	Xiōngxiāng
SP 9	Yīnlíngquán	SP 20	Zhōuróng
SP 10	Xuèhǎi	SP 21	Dàbāo
SP 11	Jīmén		

Points of Heart Meridian, **HT.**
Shǒushàoyīn Xīnjīng xué

HT 1	Jíquán	HT 6	Yīnxì
HT 2	Qīnglíng	HT 7	Shénmén
HT 3	Shàohǎi	HT 8	Shàofǔ
HT 4	Língdào	HT 9	Shàochōng
HT 5	Tōnglǐ		

Points of Small Intestine Meridian, SI.
Shǒutàiyáng Xiǎochángjīng xué

SI 1	Shàozé	SI 11	Tiānzōng
SI 2	Qiángǔ	SI 12	Bǐngfēng
SI 3	Hòuxī	SI 13	Qūyuán
SI 4	Wàngǔ	SI 14	Jiānwàishū
SI 5	Yánggǔ	SI 15	Jiānzhōngshū
SI 6	Yǎnglǎo	SI 16	Tiānchuāng
SI 7	Zhīzhèng	SI 17	Tiānróng
SI 8	Xiǎohǎi	SI 18	Quánliáo
SI 9	Jiānzhēn	SI 19	Tīnggōng
SI 10	Nàoshū		

Points of Bladder Meridian, BL.
Zútàiyáng Pángguāngjīng xué

BL 1	Jīngmíng	BL 10	Tiānzhù
BL 2	Cuánzhú(Zǎnzhú)	BL 11	Dàzhù
BL 3	Méichōng	BL 12	Fēngmén
BL 4	Qūchā(Qūchāi)	BL 13	Fèishū
BL 5	Wǔchù	BL 14	Juéyīnshū
BL 6	Chéngguāng	BL 15	Xīnshū
BL 7	Tōngtiān	BL 16	Dūshū
BL 8	Luòquè	BL 17	Géshū
BL 9	Yùzhěn	BL 18	Gānshū

BL 19	Dǎnshū	BL 44	Shéntáng
BL 20	Píshū	BL 45	Yìxǐ
BL 21	Wèishū	BL 46	Géguān
BL 22	Sānjiāoshū	BL 47	Húnmén
BL 23	Shènshū	BL 48	Yánggāng
BL 24	Qìhǎishū	BL 49	Yìshè
BL 25	Dàchángshū	BL 50	Wèicāng
BL 26	Guānyuánshū	BL 51	Huāngmén
BL 27	Xiǎochángshū	BL 52	Zhìshì
BL 28	Pángguāngshū	BL 53	Bāohuāng
BL 29	Zhōnglǚshū	BL 54	Zhìbiān
BL 30	Báihuánshū	BL 55	Héyáng
BL 31	Shàngliáo	BL 56	Chéngjīn
BL 32	Cìliáo	BL 57	Chéngshān
BL 33	Zhōngliáo	BL 58	Fēiyáng
BL 34	Xiàliáo	BL 59	Fūyáng
BL 35	Huìyáng	BL 60	Kūnlún
BL 36	Chéngfú	BL 61	Púcān(Púshēn)
BL 37	Yīnmén	BL 62	Shēnmài
BL 38	Fúxì	BL 63	Jīnmén
BL 39	Wěiyáng	BL 64	Jīnggǔ
BL 40	Wěizhōng	BL 65	Shùgǔ
BL 41	Fùfén	BL 66	Zútōnggǔ
BL 42	Pòhù	BL 67	Zhìyīn
BL 43	Gāohuāng		

Points of Kidney Meridian, **KI.**
Zúshǎoyīn Shènjīng xué

KI 1	Yǒngquán	KI 15	Zhōngzhù
KI 2	Rángǔ	KI 16	Huāngshū
KI 3	Tàixī	KI 17	Shāngqū
KI 4	Dàzhōng	KI 18	Shíguān
KI 5	Shuǐquán	KI 19	Yīndū
KI 6	Zhàohǎi	KI 20	Fùtōnggǔ
KI 7	Fùliū	KI 21	Yōumén
KI 8	Jiāoxìn	KI 22	Bùláng
KI 9	Zhùbīn	KI 23	Shénfēng
KI 10	Yīngǔ	KI 24	Língxū
KI 11	Hénggǔ	KI 25	Shéncáng
KI 12	Dàhè	KI 26	Yùzhōng
KI 13	Qìxué	KI 27	Shūfú
KI 14	Sìmǎn		

Points of Pericardium Meridian, **PC.**
Shǒujuéyīn Xīnbāojīng xué

PC 1	Tiānchí	PC 6	Nèiguān
PC 2	Tiānquán	PC 7	Dàlíng
PC 3	Qūzé	PC 8	Láogōng
PC 4	Xìmén	PC 9	Zhōngchōng
PC 5	Jiānshǐ		

Points of Triple Energizer Meridian, TE.
Shǒushàoyáng Sānjiāojīng xué

TE 1	Guānchōng	TE 13	Nàohuì
TE 2	Yèmén	TE 14	Jiānliáo
TE 3	Zhōngzhǔ	TE 15	Tiānliáo
TE 4	Yángchí	TE 16	Tiānyǒu
TE 5	Wàiguān	TE 17	Yìfēng
TE 6	Zhīgōu	TE 18	Chìmài(Qìmài)
TE 7	Huìzōng	TE 19	Lúxī
TE 8	Sānyángluò	TE 20	Jiǎosūn
TE 9	Sìdú	TE 21	Ěrmén
TE 10	Tiānjǐng	TE 22	Ěrhéliáo *
TE 11	Qīnglěngyuān		Héliáo§
TE 12	Xiāoluò	TE 23	Sīzhúkōng

* § Either of these can be used.

Points of Gallbladder Meridian, GB.
Zúshàoyáng Dǎnjīng xué

GB 1	Tóngzǐliáo	GB 9	Tiānchōng
GB 2	Tīnghuì	GB 10	Fúbái
GB 3	Shàngguān	GB 11	Tóuqiàoyīn
GB 4	Hànyàn	GB 12	Wángǔ
GB 5	Xuánlú	GB 13	Běnshén
GB 6	Xuánlí	GB 14	Yángbái
GB 7	Qūbīn	GB 15	Tóulínqì
GB 8	Shuàigǔ	GB 16	Mùchuāng

GB 17	Zhèngyíng	GB 31	Fēngshì
GB 18	Chénglíng	GB 32	Zhōngdú
GB 19	Nǎokōng	GB 33	Xīyángguān
GB 20	Fēngchí	GB 34	Yánglíngquán
GB 21	Jiānjǐng	GB 35	Yángjiāo
GB 22	Yuānyè	GB 36	Wàiqiū
GB 23	Zhéjīn	GB 37	Guāngmíng
GB 24	Rìyuè	GB 38	Yángfǔ
GB 25	Jīngmén	GB 39	Xuánzhōng
GB 26	Dàimài	GB 40	Qiūxū
GB 27	Wǔshū	GB 41	Zúlínqì
GB 28	Wéidào	GB 42	Dìwǔhuì
GB 29	Jūliáo	GB 43	Xiáxī
GB 30	Huántiào	GB 44	Zúqiàoyīn

Points of Liver Meridian, **LR.**
Zújuéyīn Gānjīng xué

LR 1	Dàdūn	LR 8	Qūquán
LR 2	Xíngjiān	LR 9	Yīnbāo
LR 3	Tàichōng	LR 10	Zúwǔlǐ
LR 4	Zhōngfēng	LR 11	Yīnlián
LR 5	Lígōu	LR 12	Jímài
LR 6	Zhōngdū	LR 13	Zhāngmén
LR 7	Xīguān	LR 14	Qīmén

Points of Governor Vessel, GV.
Dūmài xué

GV 1	Chángqiáng	GV 15	Yǎmén
GV 2	Yāoshū	GV 16	Fēngfǔ
GV 3	Yāoyángguān	GV 17	Nǎohù
GV 4	Mìngmén	GV 18	Qiángjiān
GV 5	Xuánshū	GV 19	Hòudǐng
GV 6	Jǐzhōng	GV 20	Bǎihuì
GV 7	Zhōngshū	GV 21	Qiándǐng
GV 8	Jīnsuō	GV 22	Xìnhuì
GV 9	Zhìyáng	GV 23	Shàngxīng
GV 10	Língtái	GV 24	Shéntíng
GV 11	Shéndào	GV 25	Sùliáo
GV 12	Shēnzhù	GV 26	Shuǐgōu
GV 13	Táodào	GV 27	Duìduān
GV 14	Dàzhuī	GV 28	Yínjiāo

Points of Conception Vessel, CV.
Rénmài xué

CV 1	Huìyīn	CV 5	Shímén
CV 2	Qūgǔ	CV 6	Qìhǎi
CV 3	Zhōngjí	CV 7	Yīnjiāo
CV 4	Guānyuán	CV 8	Shénquè

CV 9	Shuǐfēn	CV 18	Yùtáng
CV 10	Xiàwǎn	CV 19	Zǐgōng
CV 11	Jiànlǐ	CV 20	Huágài
CV 12	Zhōngwǎn	CV 21	Xuánjī
CV 13	Shàngwǎn	CV 22	Tiāntū
CV 14	Jùquè	CV 23	Liánquán
CV 15	Jiūwěi	CV 24	Chéngjiāng
CV 16	Zhōngtíng		
CV 17	Tánzhōng		
	(Shànzhōng)		

Extra Points of Head and Neck, HN.
Tóujǐng xué

Ex-HN 1	Sìshéncōng	Ex-HN 9	Nèiyíngxiāng
* Ex-HN 2	Dāngyáng	Ex-HN 10	Jùquán
Ex-HN 3	Yìntáng	Ex-HN 11	Hǎiquán
Ex-HN 4	Yúyāo	Ex-HN 12	Jīnjīn
Ex-HN 5	Tàiyáng	* Ex-HN 13	Yùyè
Ex-HN 6	Ěrjiān	* Ex-HN 14	Yìmíng
* Ex-HN 7	Qiúhòu	* Ex-HN 15	Jǐngbǎiláo
* Ex-HN 8	Shàngyíngxiāng		

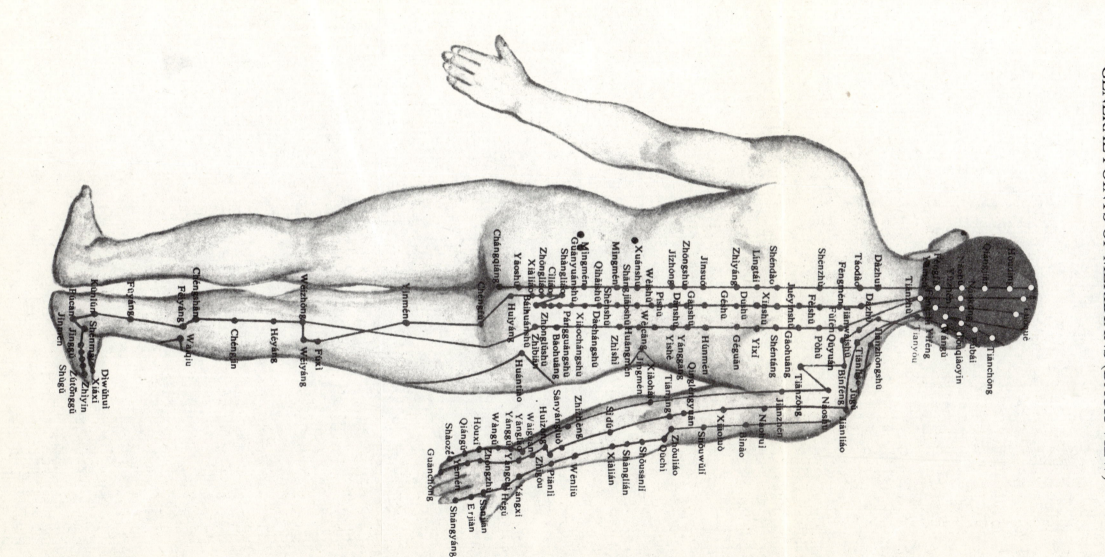

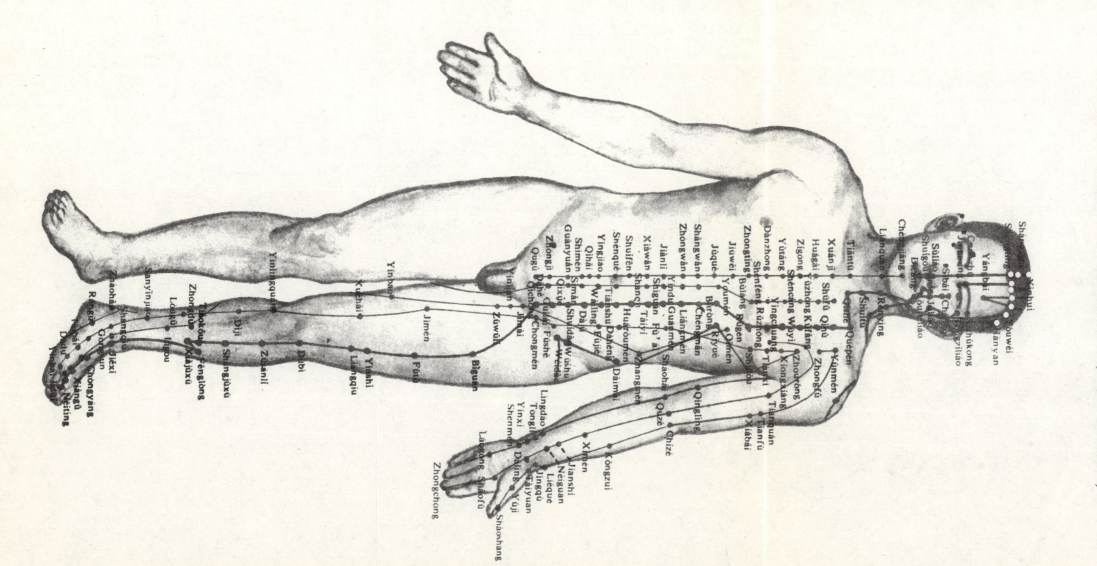

QUANSHEN JINGXUE(ZHENGMIAN)

GENERAL POINTS OF MERIDIANS (FRONT VIEW)

Extra Points of Chest and Abdomen, CA.
Xiōngfù xué

Ex-CA 1   Zǐgōng

Extra Points of Back, B.
Bèibù xué

* Ex-B 1	Dìngchuǎn	* Ex-B 6	Yāoyí
Ex-B 2	Jiájǐ	Ex-B 7	Yáoyǎn
* Ex-B 3	Wèiwǎnxiàshū	Ex-B 8	Shíqīzhuī
Ex-B 4	Pǐgēn	Ex-B 9	Yāoqí
* Ex-B 5	Xiàzhìshì		

Extra Points of Upper Extremities, UE.
Shàngzhī xué

Ex-UE 1	Zhǒujiān	* Ex-UE 7	Yāotòngdiǎn
Ex-UE 2	Erbái	* Ex-UE 8	Wàiláogōng
Ex-UE 3	Zhōngquán	Ex-UE 9	Bāxié
Ex-UE 4	Zhōngkuí	Ex-UE 10	Sìfèng
Ex-UE 5	Dàgǔkōng	Ex-UE 11	Shíxuān
Ex-UE 6	Xiǎogǔkōng		

Extra Points of Lower Extremities, **LE.**
Xiàzhī xué

* Ex-LE 1 Kuāngǔ
Ex-LE 2 Hèdǐng
* Ex-LE 3 Xīnèi
* Ex-LE 4 Nèixīyǎn

Ex-LE 5 Xīyǎn
Ex-LE 6 Dǎnnáng

* Ex-LE 7 Lánwěi
Ex-LE 8 Nèihuáijiān
Ex-LE 9 Wàihuáijiān
Ex-LE 10 Bāfēng
Ex-LE 11 Dúyīn
* Ex-LE 12 Qìduān

* Selected at the meeting in Hong Kong in 1985, the other 31 being selected at teh meeting in Tokyo in 1984.

图书在版编目(CIP)数据

常见病气功疗法:英文/李向明,燕山主编;余敏等译.
北京:学苑出版社,1997.11
ISBN 7 – 5077 – 0111 – 5

Ⅰ.常⋯ Ⅱ.①李⋯ ②燕⋯ ③余⋯ Ⅲ.常见病 – 气功
疗法 Ⅳ.R247.4

中国版本图书馆CIP数据核字(97)第16837号

常见病气功疗法

李向明 燕山主编

余敏 陆小贞 王芳 林焕英 译

学苑出版社出版
(中国北京万寿路西街11号)
邮政编码100036
北京仰山印刷厂印刷
中国国际图书贸易总公司发行
(中国北京车公庄西路35号)
北京邮政信箱第399号 邮政编码100044
32开本 英文版 1997年11月第1版第1次印刷
ISBN 7 – 5077 – 0111 – 5/R·22
02800
14 – E – 3189P

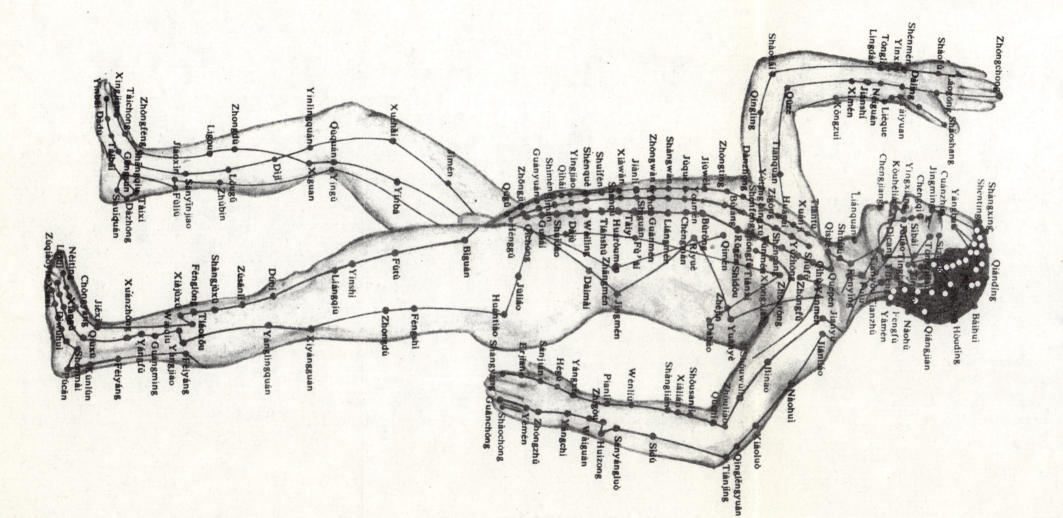

QUANSHEN JINGXUE(CEMIAN)
GENERAL POINTS OF MERIDIANS (SIDE VIEW)